Power Over Pornography

The Breakthrough Formula for Overcoming
Pornography Addiction

Brian Brandenburg

ISBN: 1484975863
ISBN 13: 9781484975862

Library of Congress Control Number: 2013909617
CreateSpace Independent Publishing Platform
North Charleston, South Carolina

Contents

Preface

Ten years ago, I attended the family weekend at the conclusion of a thirty-day intensive drug rehabilitation for a family member with a drug addiction. The out-of-state facility had an excellent reputation.

The purpose of the family weekend was to help family and close friends learn how to help the person without being an enabler. I learned about the signs of drug and alcohol addiction and the treatments. Until I attended the three-day weekend, I didn't realize how little I knew about how to help addicts.

I could provide much more detail about the path that led to my family member's addiction, treatment, and so forth, but that is not the reason I'm sharing this experience with you. On the first day of parents' weekend, one of the leaders of the program spoke to us. His eye patch, tattoos, unkempt hair, and large stature were intimidating, but he spoke with authenticity and sincerity.

He was an alcoholic who was nineteen years sober. He told us that his program and a few like it throughout the country were recognized as the best drug and alcohol rehab facilities in the nation and the world. He spoke proudly of their status as a twelve-step program and explained how twelve-step programs are proven to be the only working way to manage addictions. He then said, "Our recidivism rate is eighty percent." He paused, and then added, "Eighty percent of those who attend our program will drink or use within one year."

He kept speaking, but I didn't hear much of the rest of his talk. He talked a little about the attendees being equipped with the knowledge and tools to recover from future relapses, but my focus was on the failure rate. My immediate thoughts were, *It's one of the best rehab programs in the country, and the best they can do is 20 percent success?* And *This place costs tens of thousands of dollars, and there's an 80 percent chance of failure?*

Despite the great deal I learned over the next few days, I couldn't get the 80 percent recidivism rate out of my mind. I thought, *There has to be a better way.* From that thought sprung ten years of search and research to find a better way. In the following pages, you'll read about and experience that way.

Several months after returning from the rehab facility's family weekend, I was invited to attend a meeting of pastors (bishops) as a substitute for my pastor. He was out of town and asked me to attend and take notes for him. One of the discussions that took place during the meeting was about the difficulty congregation members had with overcoming the addiction to viewing pornography. The pastors discussed various ways of helping, including prayer, scripture study, attendance at twelve-step addiction recovery programs, and more, but no one seemed to have a solution for the inevitable series of relapses.

By this time, my research had led me to read many books and articles. Most of these had a nugget or two of value but no solution to the problem of relapse, either with pornography or drugs and alcohol. I was discouraged but determined. My search was focused on results. In fact, I was open to a variety of treatment methods if they produced better results.

In the meantime, I was asked to serve as pastor of my congregation. In addition to other duties, I began helping people overcome addictions as part of my role. Just as it was discussed at the meeting, I discovered that a pornography addiction was the most difficult for people to overcome; it was also the least researched and least discussed form of addiction, with the fewest effective options available that pastors could use to help others.

My interest in a cure—or at least better treatment programs—continued growing even stronger over the next several years. I discovered parts of programs that worked and implemented those methods right away, but I usually found holes in them too. As I've continued my on-the-job training and research over the past four years, I've developed a comprehensive treatment method and system that results in roughly 80 percent success rates, much higher than I've seen in any other program. I've recently implemented the follow-up methods included in this book, and I hope they will boost the success rate even higher.

I'll plan to continue to monitor success rates. For now, I take great satisfaction in seeing longtime addicts free of their pornography addictions and feeling happier and freer than they've felt in years. I rejoice in seeing young married men free of the guilt, shame, and suffering that pornography brings. They thought marriage would solve their addiction but discovered that it didn't. I'm grateful to see adolescents and early twentysomethings get back on track with their relationships, their levels of confidence, and their performances at work and school as a result of being porn-free.

I feel obligated to share this system with as many people as possible, so that they can be free of their pornography addictions and the terrible toll this addiction takes on their lives and the lives of their loved ones. I hope you benefit by the methods and the system presented in the following pages. When you are experiencing freedom from pornography addiction, I invite you to share your story, so others may benefit, at www.poweroverpornography.com/shareyourstory.

Introduction

You are about to embark on a journey to freedom from pornography addiction and the awful consequences that this addiction brings. You'll discover principles within the Power over Pornography system that take the power away from viewing pornography and give it back to you. I think you'll be surprised at how easy the principles are to implement.

Power over Pornography is not a twelve-step program. It stands on its own. However, we think highly of twelve-step programs and believe they can be effectively used in conjunction with Power over Pornography. This is also not solely a self-discipline program. We believe that you'll experience a greater chance of success with this program; it requires the self-discipline to read and implement simple exercises, but it does not rely on increased self-discipline while dealing with the temptation to view pornography.

Power over Pornography, a step-by-step recovery program, is just as effective at taking back your power over masturbation, a behavior that often accompanies pornography viewing but can be an addiction by itself.

Power over Pornography is solution-focused, not problem-focused. We believe you primarily want to know the way to overcome your pornography addiction and are less interested in knowing why you're addicted or how you became addicted. By following the steps outlined in this book, you'll have the solution you are seeking.

While focused on solutions, Power over Pornography is not for everyone. If you have deep psychological issues or are involved in illegal activity, we recommend you consult a therapist or a lawyer.

This book is written in story form, relying upon the example of one person addicted to pornography going through the process of taking his power back with the help of an expert guide. We hope this facilitates your learning.

You'll also see homework assignments after most chapters. The homework is easy but important. It will solidify the concepts and the steps and assist you in implementing them. Please complete the homework for the best results.

You'll be surprised at the discoveries you make with each chapter as you begin regaining power. You'll learn a brand new perspective that will have you asking, "Why didn't I think of that?"

Welcome to this opportunity to finally overcome your pornography addiction. Now, let's get started.

CHAPTER 1:

Is There Hope for Recovery from Pornography Addiction?

"Don't worry if you fail. Eighty percent of twelve-step participants don't succeed the first time," said the speaker. Jason was tired of failing. His church leader had told him the twelve-step program was the best recovery program for pornography addicts. *How could it be the best if it has such a high failure rate?* he thought. *Is there no way for me to overcome this addiction?*

Jason felt hopeless. At thirty-seven years old with three children, he desperately wanted to overcome his pornography addiction. But no matter what he tried, he kept sliding back into it. His wife had recently confronted him about the pornographic websites someone had visited on the family computer. Jason suggested their ten-year-old son, Mike, visited the websites and that he would talk to him. He was embarrassed and ashamed that he was covering up his addiction by blaming his son.

As an experienced computer user, Jason also felt stupid for not deleting the website history. A long-term pornography addict, he was used to covering his tracks. He vowed to be more careful about concealing his habit, but he felt shame that he was thinking about his carelessness instead of focusing on overcoming his addiction.

Just nine months ago, he had completed a twelve-step program that his wife didn't know he was attending. The experienced twelve-steppers advised him to tell his wife as part of his recovery, but Jason was too afraid of her reaction. Would she leave him or look at him as a failure? Would she ever want to be with him again?

So he continued attending the program without her knowledge, and it worked! Jason was elated to be free of his addiction. He gradually felt more love come back into his life, and he smiled more. His relationship with his wife and children improved. He felt more joy than he had felt in years.

He wasn't sure how it happened, but he reverted back to his old habits after six months. Granted, this was the longest he had refrained from viewing pornography. But, after one moment of weakness late at night, he was back into the same pattern that made his life miserable for so long.

"Let's take a ten-minute break."

This statement broke into Jason's thoughts, and he realized that he hadn't heard the last thirty minutes of the meeting. He was disheartened to be back and to learn that he wasn't alone in returning to his pornography addiction. He was back at this twelve-step meeting to begin again, and he was discouraged at the statistics on recidivism that the speaker mentioned. The hopelessness that had accompanied him for so many years returned.

At the break, Jason stayed inside, while over half the attendees walked outside for some fresh air. Some of the others moved to the back of the room for a snack or some water. Jason didn't feel like interacting with anyone, so he stayed in his seat, wallowing in his hopelessness.

"Hi, I'm David." Jason looked up to see a large man with graying blond hair. He appeared to be in his early sixties, and there was kindness in his smile. Jason saw his outstretched hand and weakly raised his hand to shake it. "I noticed you weren't joining the others, so I thought I would come over and say hi."

Jason perked up a little to know that someone had noticed him.

David continued. "I couldn't help but notice that you look a bit disappointed. I haven't seen you here for a few months, but I remember the last time you shared. I could tell you were changed as you described how happy you were as a result of your twelve-step journey. I hate to jump to conclusions, but you don't look the same. Have you relapsed?"

Jason wasn't comfortable talking about his addiction and relapse for fear of his wife, family, friends, or colleagues finding out. He couldn't imagine the shame he would feel if that happened. But he believed that the twelve-step meetings were safe and that the people there kept things in confidence. He confided more to the strangers during these meetings than to anyone close to him.

Jason vaguely recognized David from before. David made Jason feel OK about sharing his weaknesses. He also seemed genuinely interested and sincere. This man's warmth made Jason instantly comfortable. Jason's first impression of David was positive, and this feeling remained after several months of not seeing him.

"I guess you could say that," Jason said. "I thought following the twelve steps was the answer. I felt like I would never relapse into my old habits after I finished the program. Now I hear that relapse is expected nearly eighty percent of the time. It's discouraging to think that there isn't a way to rid myself of my addiction once and for all."

Jason opened up and said more than he thought he would. "I know I'm supposed to tell my wife and loved ones about my addiction and get their support, but I just can't bring myself to do it. I'm afraid my wife will leave me. She's very religious—we both are—and I don't think she would stand for it." He felt embarrassed admitting he was religious.

"It's usually a good idea to tell your loved ones, but I understand your concern about her reaction." The look in David's eyes conveyed his sympathy.

Jason responded, "I'm afraid she'll find out if I come to the meetings regularly again. Even though I'm afraid of her reaction, I'm also deeply ashamed and humiliated that I'm not strong enough to overcome this. I don't want to admit that to her."

"Why don't you try continuing in the program without telling her? Then when you feel the time is right, you can begin talking about it with her."

"When I completed the program last fall, I told her it was a special continuing education requirement for work. I don't think she'll buy it this time." Jason felt that the excuse he had given his wife was half-true. His addiction was hurting his work performance. Colleagues who started their careers at the same time he did were being promoted, but he had stayed in the same position for the last four years. Despite this plateau, he was used to good performance reviews; however, his last one was mediocre, and he was fearful of losing his job. He knew his pornography habit was impacting his work performance.

Jason explained, "Becky wasn't happy about my missing family time two evenings per week, but she understood because it was only for a few months. I don't like the idea of deceiving her anymore. For a while, I thought I was no longer in love with her, but once I was free of my addiction, my love for her returned gradually but strongly. I feel like I will hurt her whether I keep deceiving her or if I tell her about my pornography addiction."

As soon as Jason said this, he recognized that he was deceiving his wife every day he looked at pornography, and he fell silent. He was afraid he had already revealed too much about himself to David. He expected David to say, "Well, it was nice to meet you, Jason. Good luck with your wife," and then quickly move away.

David met Jason's eyes and didn't say anything for a few seconds. Jason felt listened to and understood. When Jason had revealed his secret addiction to his pastor before initially attending the twelve-step program, he was not greeted with this level of understanding.

Jason had struggled for years before making an appointment to confess this to the head of his congregation to seek advice and help. When he finally mustered up the courage, he was greeted with a rebuke—done in love—instead of the understanding he expected.

His pastor told him how the addiction would destroy his family and that he just needed to stop. He would receive heavenly help if he sincerely prayed and fasted about it, and he would be able to overcome the addiction.

Jason had already tried for years to call upon the powers of heaven to help him; he felt that he had received that power from time to time, even refraining from looking at pornography for months at a time on occasion. He had fasted and prayed deeply and sincerely, but he always reverted back to viewing pornography.

He followed his pastor's advice to install Internet filters on his computer and to locate the computer in a central area so that anyone could walk by and see what was on the screen. This helped temporarily, but when everyone else was asleep, he viewed pornography on certain sites that escaped the filters.

When he saw a twelve-step addiction recovery program on his church website, Jason was intrigued. He heard about Alcoholics Anonymous and knew it was the genesis of twelve-step programs. He remembered that it had a long history and a good reputation for helping people overcome addictions.

Jason recalled how difficult it was to decide to attend his first twelve-step meeting. He had denied for years that he was addicted to pornography, claiming to himself that he could stop if he really wanted to, but he didn't really want to. He thought it wasn't so bad if no one knew about it. Besides, Becky didn't want to have sex as often as he did, and pornography provided an outlet for his more powerful sex drive. As he thought about these rationalizations now, he realized they were just excuses that prolonged his addiction.

When he finally realized that his excuses were not helping him and that his addiction threatened his marriage, career, and family, he decided to try a twelve-step sexual addiction program. Jason deliberately chose not to attend the program sponsored by his church; he attended a program far from home and work. He didn't want to risk his family, friends, or church associates finding out about his attendance.

Jason loved the program. He felt that it reflected a strong understanding of the power of addiction. He was gratified to know that he was not the only one struggling against his addiction with little success. When he admitted that he was powerless over his addiction, he felt hopeful that he could recover. That hope blossomed, and Jason remained "sober" from his pornography addiction for six months, as mentioned previously.

He knew he was supposed to continue attending meetings to remain porn-free, but he also felt he was healed of his addiction and couldn't spend any more time away from his wife, kids, or job. He would have to manage without meetings.

Jason enjoyed life more during those six months than he had in years. He didn't fully realize the joy he was experiencing until he looked back over the six-month period. During the first few months, he faced numerous trials and concluded that overcoming the addiction had not resulted in a tremendous improvement in his life. But near the end of the six months, the transformation became crystal clear. He felt greater love for his wife and kids, and it also seemed like he was performing better at work. Jason felt like he was more in tune spiritually than he had been since before his teens. Life seemed good again.

As he reflected on the addiction-free time, he realized how damaging pornography had been to his life and relationships and how much better his life was without it. The anger directed at his wife and kids went away almost miraculously. He had not associated the anger with his pornography habit until he was able to see the difference in his life firsthand.

"I'm sorry about your relapse and discouragement," David whispered. I'm also a pornography addict. I've been sober for twenty-two years, and I may be able to help you."

Jason shifted his focus toward David. "I'm not sure there is help for me if I don't attend these meetings on a regular basis."

David gently responded, "I still receive strength from the twelve-step meetings—otherwise I wouldn't be here—but I've discovered some principles and practices that go beyond the twelve-step addiction recovery program. They have helped me remain free of my pornography addiction. If you feel like they may help you, I'd be happy to share them with you."

Jason felt a little hope returning. He didn't know David very well, but he sensed David's sincerity and believed he wanted to help. The hope was fleeting. Jason's inner skeptic prompted him to blurt out, "How much does it cost?" He felt bad the minute he asked the question but didn't want to appear naïve. He also wasn't prepared to spend money earmarked for his family on an expensive treatment program.

David didn't blink. He met Jason's skepticism with a sincere answer. "It will only cost you some of your time. I'm willing to help you so that you can help someone else. I believe that's one of the silver linings of my addiction. Former addicts can empathize and help others climb out of a personal abyss.

"I believe you'll be able to help many others move from a life of addiction to a life of love and joy. One of my great satisfactions in life is to see hard-core addicts become loving husbands and fathers, to see hopeless people begin to experience a hope and love that they thought was lost and to see their work lives progress even beyond their ambitions."

David's statement conveyed peace and warmth, and a little more hope returned to Jason's heart. Before Jason could reply, the facilitator spoke from the front of the room. "Let's take our seats and get started." Jason briefly turned toward the facilitator. When he turned back, David was returning to his own seat. Jason wanted to rush after him but remained seated for the rest of the meeting.

He couldn't remember much of what was said during the rest of the meeting, but he sensed a spirit of healing in the room. He kept thinking about his short conversation with David and the hope and peace that it brought to him. He determined to meet with David and learn more about the principles and practices that gave David strength and power over his addiction.

CHAPTER 2:

Am I Addicted to Pornography?

As Jason drove home, the hope he had felt in the meeting stayed with him, replacing his shame and hopelessness. He felt like David had come into his life at the right time. Maybe his prayers were finally being answered, and this would be the way out of his porn addiction.

He smiled as he thought about David's gentle way, his lack of judgment, and his sincerity in wanting to help. Before the twelve-step program, Jason had tried a couple of recovery programs for Internet addiction and tried many other ways to overcome his pornography addiction without success.

Jason first viewed pornography as an eleven-year-old. He remembered the day it happened, twenty-six years ago, when he was walking home after school. He saw a group of his friends stopped on the trail that went through the woods on the way home. He caught up to them and asked what they were doing.

"You gotta see this," one of his friends replied. Jason looked closer and saw a magazine opened to a photo of a naked woman. He felt it was wrong, but he kept looking as one of the boys turned the pages, showing more photos of this woman and others. That night he couldn't get the photos out of his mind and wanted to see them again.

Jason had recently learned that eleven is the average age that young people are exposed to pornography. Until then, he had always thought it was unusual that he viewed it at such a young age. Although he didn't get the chance to view pornography often during middle school, he acquired his own magazines in high school and then switched to the Internet for viewing pornography.

He never thought he was addicted; he was just enjoying looking at pictures of naked ladies. Sometimes he went weeks and months without viewing pornography, thinking he could stop when he wanted to. But he always went back to it.

As Jason drove, he thought, *I became addicted when I was eleven years old, but I didn't realize it until last year.* He felt foolish as this thought hit him. *I've learned what it means to be addicted, and I'm glad I'm finally doing something about it. I wish I would have done that many, many years ago. I thought the problem would go away as I got older, when I got married or when I had less stress in my life.*

Now I know that the problem doesn't get better on its own. I would have been way better off if I had addressed it many years ago. I know it doesn't help to dwell on the past, so I'll just be grateful I'm finally doing something about it. I've been stupid to live with pornography for so long.

As Jason neared home, he reflected deeply on his addiction. *I've been trying to tell myself that I wasn't addicted because I could go long stretches without viewing pornography and could quit when I wanted. I now realize those are lies, and I knew in my heart all along that they were lies.*

Now I know that frequency, intensity, and duration don't matter in defining addiction for me. Viewing pornography is bad for me, bad for my family, and bad for my work. I'm addicted even if I view pornography only once a year.

If I know that I don't want to do it but I do it anyway, even infrequently, then I'm not living according to my own values and standards, so I'm addicted. In essence, when I look at pornography, I'm doing something I really don't want to do. To me, that's the definition of addiction, and I don't want it anymore.

Jason felt he was finally willing to admit the truth to himself about his pornography viewing, and he felt that this change could only help as he tried David's principles and practices. He smiled as his thoughts turned from the past to the present. *It's about time. I think this is going to help, so I'm going to try it.*

CHAPTER 3:

The Power of Commitment

"Jason, I need that reconciliation by the end of the day." As an accountant, Jason wasn't used to having deadlines reiterated. However, he had missed a few deadlines during the past few weeks, so he understood why his boss, Bruce, was now focused on the deadline.

After Jason was free of his addiction for six months and then went back to it, he saw clearly that his work performance improved while he was free of pornography and slid when he wasn't.

He wasn't sure if it was an absolute cause-and-effect connection or if his late nights looking at pornography led to sleep deprivation, which then led to poor performance. He also considered the possibility that he was behind because his colleagues focused on improving their work-related knowledge or simply did more work during the time he spent looking at pornography.

One other thought occurred to him. He knew his self-confidence was markedly higher and his step was lighter when he was temporarily not viewing pornography. He now recognized that his confidence dropped when he was not porn-free, so he tied this change directly to viewing pornography. Jason also knew that a person's confidence is reflected in everything they do and in every interaction they have. *So*, he thought, *my pornography viewing must be impacting my performance and everyone's perception of my leadership abilities.*

Jason realized that the pornography addiction resulted in feelings of shame. He felt this shame because he resolved every day to stop but still viewed pornography, because he was violating his marriage vows, and because he was spending his time viewing pornography instead of taking care of his family. It had to be impacting his job performance. Regardless of the reasons and results, Jason was convinced that pornography was hurting his performance on the job.

"I'm right on schedule and should have it to you by four thirty." Jason wanted to beat the deadline for two reasons: to show Bruce that he still had it and to make sure he wasn't late for his first meeting with David. He was curious about the principles and practices that could finally provide a way out of his addiction.

He was hopeful but still a little skeptical. He worried that the program was just another self-improvement program telling him to discipline himself better. He felt hopeless at improving his self-discipline and greeted self-improvement programs with cynicism. *They work best for the person charging money for them* he thought.

At 4:25 p.m., Jason handed the completed reconciliation to his boss. Bruce acted a bit surprised when he took it. He smiled at Jason and then turned back toward his computer. Jason knew he was interrupting Bruce's work, so he didn't linger, but he felt satisfied with Bruce's smile. As Jason turned to leave, he felt a little lighter. He smiled to himself as he exited the office.

Jason pulled his car up to the address David had given him. It was a beautiful, simply landscaped colonial house in a nice neighborhood about eleven miles from Jason's house. Jason felt a twinge of guilt about coming to David's house.

When David suggested they meet at a restaurant near Jason's workplace, Jason said he was still worried about others finding out about his addiction and preferred to meet in a more private setting. David quickly volunteered his own home.

"I have a private office in my home. I want you to be able to focus on learning, not on wondering who may be watching."

Jason feigned objection but quickly accepted when David insisted. He was happy to be meeting in a place where his addiction was not likely to be discovered by others but felt his quick acceptance may seem like imposing on David.

Before Jason rang the doorbell, David opened the door, greeting Jason with a warm handshake. "Welcome, Jason. I hope you didn't have any problem finding my home."

"No, your directions were great. Thanks again for letting me come here. I hope it's not hard on you or your family."

"Not at all. I'm glad we can meet here. We have a little more control over the environment, but I apologize in advance that we may be interrupted from time to time." David motioned towards the hallway, "When I'm home, I'm fair game for family interruptions."

David motioned for Jason to come in and waved his hand toward the door on the right. Jason felt a peaceful spirit in David's house. Somehow he had expected this. It reflected the peace he felt when he first talked with David at the twelve-step meeting. As he entered David's office, the peaceful feeling stayed.

"Please sit down. I know you're pressed for time to get to your family tonight, so let's dive right into action.

"I have a whiteboard in the office so we can record some of the most important concepts. If you're anything like me, concepts stay with you more when you see them as well as hear them. In fact, the more senses we use in learning, the more we'll retain.

"Jason, are you familiar with the concept of different learning styles?"

"I'm not sure what you mean."

"Some people learn better by reading, while some learn better by listening; others learn better by watching, and still others learn by participating. Some people need a combination of all these methods. Does that sound familiar?"

"Oh, yeah. I've learned about that in school and on the job. I tend to be a reader, but I'm OK at absorbing knowledge other ways as well."

"Great, then using a combination won't slow down your learning, and it should help you remember and apply the key concepts better."

"Thanks. Learning in different ways keeps me from getting bored."

David chuckled and said, "I hope you won't get too bored with what you're going to learn. In a few moments, you'll be learning the keys to gaining power over pornography in ways that you've never thought of. The concepts will ring true, but their application will be new to you.

"You'll be able to overcome the addiction without feeling deprived."

Jason interrupted. "You mean by learning the self-discipline to deny myself, I can overcome the addiction?" He couldn't hold back his skepticism.

Jason was used to facing annoyed looks when he expressed his skepticism, but David seemed to take it in stride, and the warmth in his eyes stayed. "We're jumping ahead of ourselves, but this is not a course in improving your self-discipline. The only discipline you'll need is to follow the program. You'll understand this better as we move along."

Jason couldn't grasp how he could possibly overcome his pornography viewing without exercising self-discipline—discipline that he lacked—but he was beginning to trust David.

David turned to the whiteboard and wrote "Priority → Commitment."

"Jason, you seem very motivated to rid yourself of your pornography addiction. But it's important that we determine if it's a major priority in your life and if you're willing to commit to follow *all* the steps required to overcome your addiction.

"Some people experience early success and quit before completing all the training and learning all the concepts. Others let the seemingly urgent priorities of life overtake the important priority of this learning, and they stop before they're finished. Some just have a strong habit of not finishing what they start. Those who don't finish their learning and training are the ones who relapse after a few weeks or months.

"I'm willing to spend my time teaching and training you, but before we begin, I want to make sure the timing is right for you and that you'll be able to finish the training and make it a priority. If you think you won't be able to finish, then we will postpone starting until you are in a better position to finish the entire course during the six-week duration. It's important to your success that you come to each session according to the schedule.

"The schedule provides for sufficient time between sessions to absorb and apply the specific concepts and exercises of that session, but it does not allow too much time to elapse. If too much time passes between sessions, the synergy of the concepts is lost, and some of the power drains out of the learning."

Jason felt like his commitment was being challenged but wasn't sure how to respond. He didn't know any details about the training and the time commitment involved. He trusted David to a point but didn't really know him that well, so he wasn't sure he was committed to the training. He wanted to try it, and then he could judge whether it was worth committing to.

David, sensing Jason's wariness, added, "I know you aren't familiar with the program yet and you don't know me that well. Let me outline the training commitment and touch on its potential impact so you can see if it's something you want to commit to."

Jason breathed a sigh of relief and vowed to do a better job of keeping his thoughts and feelings from being revealed in his facial expressions.

Turning to the board, David wrote: "Fourteen sessions of thirty to forty minutes each plus outside homework of ten to thirty minutes per session." Underneath this statement, he wrote: "Six weeks."

"I've found from teaching others that the ideal time frame for the training is six weeks. Early on, we will meet three times per week, and near the end of the training, we will meet twice per week for a total of fourteen sessions.

"I want to emphasize again that it's important before you start the training that you commit to finishing it."

Jason was ready to commit even though he didn't know much about the program. He felt good about David, and he figured that committing ten to fourteen total hours over six weeks for a chance to overcome a decades-long addiction was worth the commitment despite his remaining skepticism.

He thought about the one concept that was still nagging him from a Stephen Covey leadership seminar he had attended several years previously. The Covey facilitator asked, "What one thing in your life, if you changed it, would make the biggest difference?" Jason knew immediately that the answer was his pornography addiction, and yet he still had it seven years later.

If he couldn't commit now to fourteen hours over a mere six weeks, then he could probably never commit. Jason thought, *This truly should be—no, this is—the most important priority because it will make the biggest difference in my life.*

However, David continued explaining the commitment. "Before you commit to this, let's go over a few ground rules." He wrote on the board: "Trust the teacher" and "Focus on the outcome."

"Although we just met recently, I sense a connection and trust between us. I'm going to ask you to extend that trust a little further. I would like you to open your mind to the training; in essence, to accept that I know what I'm doing as your guide through the program and that you will greet the sessions with an open mind and will.

"I tend to be a bit cynical about new approaches, especially if they hold out the promise that I can accomplish something I'm not sure I believe. I tend to not open my mind to the new approach. Instead, I try to poke holes in it instead of listening for the purpose of learning.

"You may not be as cynical as I am, but just in case, I'm asking you to not take the cynical approach. If you find yourself becoming cynical, try dropping your cynicism momentarily when you feel it, and commit yourself to listening, learning, and applying the training with an open mind. You'll find out soon enough if it works. If you hang onto your cynical self, you may not experience the program enough to let it work for you."

Jason recognized himself in David's words. Even though he understood and agreed with David, he hesitated, worried that the training may be something weird, like hypnosis or primal therapy. He had seen a news special on the yelling therapy method and thought it was ridiculous.

David continued, reacting to Jason's hesitation. "Don't worry. It's not a fringe program. As you participate in it, you'll find it uses run-of-the-mill teaching styles. You may even find it boring, but I don't think you will."

Jason thought, *Either he can read minds, or I'm wearing my thoughts on my face.*

"Now, let's turn to the second phrase, 'Focus on the outcome,' and discuss why this should be a priority and a major commitment for you. Much of the early part of the training will be focused on consequences and outcomes, but if you don't believe the outcome is worth the effort, then your commitment will not be sufficient to finish the program.

"People with addictions make up many reasons justifying why the outcome of holding on to their addiction is not all that bad. Their rationalizations make it difficult for them to finish a program."

Jason's commitment had started to build as David spoke. "I'm very motivated. This addiction has been with me since before I was a teenager, and it's slowly destroying my life and my family. Although, like you, I tend to approach things skeptically, I'll try to drop my guard for six weeks to see if I can benefit. If this program can work to help me overcome my addiction, I sense that it will help my entire life. I can't think of a higher priority right now, even though I'm busy at work and at home.

"I've been through all the rationalizations before about how pornography is not that bad, everyone seems to be doing it, or it doesn't impact my life, and I recognize that those are lies. I'm sad that it's taken me such a long time to realize this, but six months of being porn-free helped me realize what I was missing. My pornography addiction is putting distance between me and my wife and kids, the most important people in my life. I may lose them if I don't overcome it."

Jason paused and noticed that he was speaking in a raised voice. Before he could continue, David spoke, wearing an understated smile. "I think you're sufficiently motivated and committed. You've raised just a few outcomes to focus on, and I think they're sufficient to cement your commitment. We'll get into more of them within the training.

"So, let's make it official," David said as he handed a Jason a blank piece of paper. "Commitments are cemented and made easier to fulfill when they are written and signed as well as verbalized. I'll ask you a few questions. Are you willing to write the questions and your answers on the page?"

"Sure. I think you're right. Ask away, and I'll write and sign."

"Jason, are you willing to finish this program as I've outlined it for you as long as you don't have any serious philosophical or religious differences with it?"

"Yes."

"Are you willing to trust the teacher?"

"Yes."

"Are you willing to focus on the outcome?"

"Yes," Jason stated as he clicked the pen to sign the document.

David interrupted his actions. "Wait. Before you sign, we have one other concept and question to cover."

David turned to the board again and wrote: "Priorities: don't let the urgent crowd out the important."

"I think your trust and the outcomes you're focused on will last and motivate you to finish the training, but I know you have a number of pressing demands on your time."

Jason recognized the use of the words "urgent" and "important" from Stephen Covey's time-management matrix. As he recalled, the matrix consisted of four quadrants: (1) unimportant and nonurgent, (2) unimportant and urgent, (3) important and urgent, and (4) important and nonurgent. He knew that effective time management involved getting rid of unimportant and nonurgent tasks and shifting more of his focus from the urgent and unimportant to the nonurgent and important quadrant.

He didn't always use this matrix in guiding his time management decisions, but he believed it was easy to let the important, non-urgent priorities take a backseat to urgent but less important priorities. Jason knew that to really make progress on life goals, committing to deliberately switch focus was vital.

David continued, "All the accountants I know have a lot of work, have a strong focus on deadlines, and have to put in long hours around tax due dates. Is that true with your job?"

"Exactly my job."

"Your wife and children are involved in the community, church, school, and other activities. My guess is that you would like to spend more time with them."

Jason nodded. "Mike just started soccer this year, and I'm the assistant coach. The season starts soon. I think it will be a blast, but it will take some of my time for practice during the week and for games on Saturdays. My wife is taking time out from her career to raise our children as a stay-at-home mom, but she volunteers a lot with church and the kids' school. She also asks me to help her or help with the kids, and I like to do that as much as I can." Jason felt a twinge of guilt; he had not helped her much lately, and her requests had decreased. Maybe she was giving up a little.

"You lead a busy life." David sympathized. "I won't get into the other demands on your time, such as your hobbies and volunteer work. You are juggling enough priorities without the addition of one more. How are you going to make this training a priority?"

Jason didn't hesitate. He had asked himself this question several times before he drove to David's house. "I typically work late two nights per week in order to get all my work done on time. To make this program a priority without jeopardizing my work performance, I plan to get to the office thirty minutes early two to three times per week, and I can work through lunch in order to spend the hours we've allocated in the late afternoons and evenings for this training. I don't plan on letting anything interfere with this priority. I sense that if it works, it can change my life more than anything else."

Dave smiled. "It's funny how easy it is for us to cruise along, knowing that we have higher priorities but not ever getting to them because we don't make time. I'm glad you've thought about this as a priority compared to the other demands on your time.

"You're correct. This program can change your life more than anything else you would prioritize. In fact, it has the potential to help you realize goals in other areas you consider priorities in your life—namely, family relationships and career progress.

"Another way of looking at it is, 'I'm not sure this is going to work for me, but it's worked for others, so I'm going to commit the ten to fourteen hours or so of initial time to see if it works for me.' This is a small time commitment when you think about the potential outcome."

Jason nodded as David switched gears. "I think you're motivated and have met the three necessary precursors to starting the program: you trust the teacher, at least so far." David smiled. "You are focused on the outcomes, and you're willing to forego urgent but less important priorities to make this a main priority.

"So, let's return to the questions. Will you continue writing down the questions and your answers?"

"Let's do it."

"Are you willing to forego urgent but less important activities to make this a priority?"

"Yes," Jason stated as he signed the document.

"Great. I think making your commitment both verbally and in writing will help you finish the program and overcome your addiction. It will also help you feel accountable. I want to make sure you have all the ingredients you need to succeed, so I'm glad we're off to a good start.

"I think the power of a written commitment will also help you overcome any obstacles along the way. Have you heard the saying, 'A goal not written is merely a wish?' Well, you've just turned a wish into a commitment. That will give you power to achieve the goal at a rate that is many times that of an unwritten commitment or goal."

MY COMMITMENT

Commitments are cemented and made easier to fulfill when they are written and signed

1. Am I willing to finish this program as outlined as long as I don't have any serious philosophical or religious differences with it?
   Yes
2. Am I willing to trust the teacher?
   Yes
3. Am I willing to focus on the outcome?
   Yes
4. Am I willing to forego urgent but less important activities to make this a priority?
   Yes

_____

(Signature)

The power of a written commitment will help you overcome obstacles faced along the way. A goal not written is merely a wish.

Note: *If you're reading this book to rid yourself of your own addiction, it is important for you to complete the same exercises as Jason. Please refer to* poweroverpornography.com/commitment *for a pre-printed commitment letter with the list of questions and a place for your commitment signature.*

Dave added, "Before we dive in, I would like your permission to change our vocabulary a little.

"I will refer to a pornography addict as a 'viewer' throughout the training. Pornography is a big word with extremely negative connotations. We will refer to the act of looking at pornography or engaging in active pornography addiction as 'viewing.'

"The act of masturbation, which accompanies pornography viewing in the majority of viewing episodes but can also be a separate addiction, we'll call 'doing.' A masturbation addict will be referred to as a 'doer.'

"Does that make sense to you?"

Jason nodded. "I like the change."

David continued by saying, "We'll also use positive references to living a life free of pornography, or viewing, and free of masturbation, or doing. We'll refer to this as 'living a loving life' or 'living a life of love.' You'll learn shortly that overcoming viewing and doing leads to a huge increase in your capacity to love and in the happiness you derive from it. In a later session, we'll also turn this ambiguous concept of love into something much more concrete.

"Although these concepts are focused on overcoming pornography and masturbation addictions—viewing and doing—they can also be applied in the case of other sexual addictions, such as sexual relationships outside of marriage, visits to strip clubs, casual sex, interactions with prostitutes, homosexual encounters, and so on.

"In helping men and women overcome their pornography addiction, I've found that some of them have these related addictions. This program always helps, but I also encourage them to get professional counseling. If you have any related sexual addictions, I encourage you to get professional help as well."

David paused, waiting for Jason's reaction. Jason had been tempted to move beyond his pornography addiction to having sex outside of marriage, but he had not done it. *I think I've been lucky that I haven't ventured beyond pornography,* Jason thought. "I don't have any other sexual addictions yet, so I think we're good to go," Jason replied.

"Then we won't focus on the other items."

David was casual in mentioning other sex addictions, but just hearing them spoken made Jason nervous. He felt himself blush.

"Are you ready to get started? During our next session, we add the power of clarity to the power of commitment."

Whiteboard – Chapter 3

Priority → Commitment

- Fourteen sessions of thirty to forty minutes each
- Outside homework of ten to thirty minutes per session
- Six weeks

Trust the teacher
Focus on the outcome
Priorities: don't let the urgent crowd out the important

CHAPTER 4:

The Power of Clarity

David turned to the whiteboard again and wrote "The power of clarity," and then he stated, "The first step in overcoming your pornography addiction is to clarify the consequences of viewing pornography."

Jason looked quizzically at David, wondering out loud, "I'm not sure I get why this is an important step. Aren't the consequences obvious?"

David gently responded, "Sometimes we think that the consequences are obvious, but this is a vital step in overcoming your addiction. I think the reason will become clear to you in a moment with a simple illustration.

"Let me outline the steps in clarifying consequences, and then we can get into why it's so powerful.

"Here is what I would like you to do.

"Start by researching pornography's negative impact and list all of the consequences you discover. Then write down the five negative consequences that you most want to leave behind. Once you've completed this, research the positive impacts that overcoming pornography will have on you and list them. Write down the five positive consequences you most desire."

David turned to the board and wrote, "Realizing the power of clarity: clear consequences." Underneath that statement, he wrote: "Five biggest negative consequences," and below that, he wrote: "Five biggest positive consequences."

Dave added, "You will probably come up with a much larger list than five in each category, but I would like you to pare each list down to that number. In a past business leadership role, I learned that most people can maintain focus on no more than five items at a time. If our business plan moved beyond five key priorities, we typically accomplished less than when we limited our focus.

"The exercise of doing this also helped us select the five goals that would have the greatest impact on our company. I'm still a believer that narrowing your focus to five key goals will result in greater accomplishment than focusing on more.

"In fact, I believe that you can't effectively focus on more than five items at a time. I'm a firm believer that you get what you focus on, and trying to focus on more than five priorities at a time means you aren't focused at all.

"I didn't mean to get into so much detail about the Rule of Five, but hopefully it's helpful to you. Let's move on.

"How do you research the negative impacts of pornography? I have some ideas, but I'm interested in your thoughts, Jason."

Jason pondered the question briefly before responding. "I think much of my research can come from personal experience. I can think of many consequences that I've suffered."

David wasn't satisfied with this. "What else?" he asked. "In order for you to clear up the cloudiness of the consequences, I think you'll need to do some outside research."

Before Jason could respond, David added, "I'm sorry, Jason. I'm moving ahead too fast and using words to describe concepts we haven't covered yet.

"I just mentioned clearing up the cloudiness of consequences without an explanation. If you'll permit me to provide a quick story, I think I can provide context that will help illustrate my point and define why this step is so important.

"Several years ago, I heard a leader in my church speak to two hundred or so youth. He was tasked with motivating them to make good moral decisions during what can be a critical time in their lives.

"Many youth and way too many adults choose short-term gratification with little regard to the long-term consequences of their behavior. However, one of the universal keys to happiness is deferring short-term gratification in favor of long-term goals.

"A simple example is a young person doing homework instead of playing a video game. When a teenager chooses to do homework on time despite the desire to play a video game, he or she chooses excelling in school and gaining knowledge; this leads to graduating from high school, going to and graduating from college, a better job, and so on.

"I believe that the choice to defer short-term gratification is made easier when the consequences of both the short-term action and the inverse long-term action are clearly delineated and stated; that is, clarified.

"The speaker made this point beautifully. He used two sticks as symbols of action and consequences. Each stick was one-inch in diameter and about two feet long.

"He wrote 'action' at one end of each dowel and 'consequences' on the other end. He painted one of the dowels lightly in gold. He then rewrote the word 'action' so that it was clearly visible but left the word consequences barely visible under the paint.

"Before showing the sticks to the youth, he told them how much he enjoyed the Indiana Jones movies that began in the 1980s. The speaker described a scene from one of the movies.

"'Indiana Jones, the hero, and his enemies are in a room filled with cups of many varieties, some jeweled and ornate and others somewhat more plain. They have succeeded in their search for the Holy Grail but are not sure which cup is the real grail and which cups are imposters. A knight is guarding the cups. If one drinks from one of the cups, the Holy Grail, he will inherit a dose of healing and immortality. If one drinks from any one of the other cups, he will die.

"'As one of Indiana Jones's enemies approaches the cups, the knight instructs him to "choose wisely." He chooses a large, fancy, ornate cup and drinks. He dies. The knight points out that "he chose unwisely."

"'Indiana Jones's father has been shot by his enemies and is dying in the next room. Indiana wants to choose the cup for his father so his father can drink from it and be healed. Indiana chooses a cup for his father. Indiana drinks from the cup to make sure it's not going to kill his father.'

"He ended the description of the movie scene at that point and held up the two sticks. He asked the youth to choose one of the sticks but to choose wisely. He asked, 'Who would choose the gold-painted stick?' About twenty-five percent of the audience members raised their hands. He asked who would choose the plain stick, and the other seventy-five percent of the teens raised their hands.

"He pointed out that they must have remembered the movie scene and learned from it. Indiana Jones had picked a plain, wooden cup and was successful in choosing wisely. His father drank from the cup and was healed.

"He explained that the gold-painted stick, although better looking, was the 'stupid stick.' He explained that whenever we choose to take an action in our lives, we are choosing the consequences of that action whether they are clear to us or not. Similarly, when we pick up the action end of the stick, we pick up the consequences end of the stick at the same time whether we mean to or not. The two are attached.

"He reviewed several moral decisions the youth would face and tried to clearly lay out the short-term and long-term consequences of their positive and negative choices. We all get hit with the stupid stick, but we are especially vulnerable in our youth.

"Sometimes we get hit with the stupid stick, meaning that the consequences appear clouded; that is, we are caught up in the moment so that we forget the consequences or ignore them. In other words, at the moment of choice, the consequences can be cloudy. But the consequences are still there, and we suffer them when we take an action.

"By deliberately clarifying the consequences before taking action, we increase our chances of choosing wisely.

"One of the keys to making moral decisions is ridding ourselves of the stupid stick—in other words, making sure we are well aware of the consequences of our actions. This is also one of the keys to overcoming a viewing or doing addiction.

"I hope that when you think of acting without regard to consequences or how painful they may be that you'll consider yourself hit by the stupid stick. That realization can help you clarify consequences and make decisions based upon them.

"I like the picture that the stupid stick paints in my mind, illustrating painted-over but very real consequences. But the actual concept is grounded in solid brain science. Without getting into a lot of detail, we have separate parts of our brain with different functions and processing methods.

"One part of our brain, the frontal lobe, is the logical area that considers consequences, both long- and short-term, as it reasons and tries to reach a logical decision. Another part of our brain, the limbic system, which is referred to by some as the reptilian brain, responds to stimulus without thinking. The response is based upon natural instinct or, more often, how we've trained that part of our brain to react to stimulus.

"We'll get into more about training our brain, and just for fun, we may continue to refer to it as clarifying cloudy consequences and trading the stupid stick for the clear-consequence stick.

"Now that you have some context about the importance of removing any cloudiness surrounding consequences, let's get back to the question of research. What other sources can you use to list the consequences of viewing pornography?"

Jason was still smiling from the mental picture of the stupid stick and how he made decisions in the past without thinking through the long-term consequences. The idea of clarifying the consequences of viewing pornography seemed a little more important now.

He replied, "I know that university-level research has been performed on the effects of pornography and that many religious organizations have published research as well. This should be easy to track down on the Internet.

"Also, many leaders of my religion and other religions have spoken about the consequences that they've seen in helping people overcome addiction to pornography."

David responded, "I think you're on the right track. I've also seen firsthand, in the people I've guided through this program, the consequences of pornography addiction and the consequences of living a loving life."

Jason asked, "Will you share your list of consequences with me? It would make it a lot easier for me to narrow mine down to five negatives and five positives if I have a starting point."

David smiled. "I'll be happy to provide you my list, but it won't have as much meaning to you as your own list does. You and I could read the same research and make completely different lists of consequences based upon what rings true to us.

"The list also takes on deeper meaning to the person making it because of his or her knowledge of the context. In other words, you'll list one point of the research you're reading, but you'll also remember the context of that point, and so it will have a deeper meaning to you than it would to me. Does that make sense?"

Jason agreed with David's point and reluctantly withdrew his request for a shortcut. "I think so. I'm familiar with the concept that the teacher learns much more than the student. I view this the same way. That is, I'm learning the material to focus it into a list, and the learning process will give added meaning to that list."

"I think you're ready to do your homework. Let's review the calendar. It's important that we schedule the next five meetings within two weeks. The concepts build upon each other, so spacing sessions too far apart will mean forgetting and relearning some of the key building blocks."

David and Jason scheduled out not only the next six meetings but also the remaining meetings. They both committed to keeping the schedule.

Homework for the Power of Clarity:

1. Reread written commitment and recommit to starting and finishing the program. Commitment leads to success.
2. Research the negative and positive consequences of viewing pornography.
3. Narrow the list of consequences to the top five negative and the top five positive ones. Write them down.
4. Schedule all of the remaining training meetings on your calendar (see example or print your own calendar at www.poweroverpornography.com/calendar):
   a. Week 1: 3 sessions—one every other day
   b. Week 2: 3 sessions—one every other day
   c. Week 3: 2 sessions equally spaced
   d. Week 4: 2 sessions equally spaced
   e. Week 5: 2 sessions equally spaced
   f. Week 6: 2 sessions equally spaced

Whiteboard – Chapter 4

The Power of Clarity
- Realizing the power of clarity: Clear consequences
  - Five biggest negative consequences
  - Five biggest positive consequences

	Sunday	Monday	Tuesday	Wednesday	Thursday	Friday	Saturday
Week 1		POP Session 1: 30 min and 30 min homework		POP Session 2: 30 min and 30 min homework		POP Session 3: 30 min and 30 min homework	
Week 2		POP Session 4: 30 min and 30 min homework		POP Session 5: 30 min and 30 min homework			POP Session 6: 30 min and 30 min homework
Week 3			POP Session 7: 30 min and 30 min homework		POP Session 8: 30 min and 30 min homework		
Week 4		POP Session 9: 30 min and 30 min homework				POP Session 10: 30 min and 30 min homework	
Week 5				POP Session 11: 30 min and 30 min homework			POP Session 12: 30 min and 30 min homework
Week 6			POP Session 13: 30 min and 30 min homework			PO Session 14: 30 min and 30 min homework	

* POP is the abbreviation for Power over Pornography

CHAPTER 5:

The Power of Clarity
Part II: Negative and Positive
Consequences

As Jason drove home after his first meeting with David, he felt some strength and optimism returning. He was excited to get started on his homework assignment. He didn't know what to expect in future discussions with David, but it seemed like things were going in a promising direction.

As Jason walked in the door, he heard noise from the kitchen. He closed the door a little loudly, hoping his kids would hear. Bailey, his four-year-old daughter, usually came running and jumped into his arms. He waited briefly, but when he didn't hear the familiar pattering of her feet, he walked toward the kitchen. As Jason walked into the kitchen, he remembered yelling at Bailey last night because she had spilled her milk and it splashed all over his suit pants. Later that night, he skipped reading to her before bed because he was still mad about the milk and was busy watching TV.

Bailey didn't turn around from coloring at her small table in the corner of the kitchen when Jason greeted her. "Hi, Mike."

Jason's son was sneaking something to eat from the cupboard and turned around quickly. "Hi, Dad," he said with little emotion in his voice.

Mike, seven years old, had asked Jason to play soccer with him last night, but Jason was too tired. He rationalized that the season would be starting soon, and then he and Mike would be able to play soccer on the practice field. Now, Mike quickly left the room and didn't even ask Jason about playing soccer tonight.

Jason's wife, Becky, stirred something in a pot on the stove, looking like her normal, emotionless self. *If she would come to life,* Jason thought, *especially in the bedroom, then my life would improve 100 percent, and I wouldn't have to resort to pornography to satisfy my urges.* He hated the way she gave him the silent treatment after he yelled at the kids. *If she would discipline them more, then I wouldn't have to yell at them. Oh well. It's another miserable night at home; I'm used to it.* Jason hugged Nicole in her high chair before walking into the family room to watch TV with Mike.

"Well, were you able to complete your homework?" David asked when Jason sat down opposite the large, cherry desk in David's home office. Two days had passed since their first session.

"It was easier than I thought it would be. I was able to come up with fifteen or twenty negative consequences of pornography viewing pretty quickly. Some of them in particular really rang true to me, like you said they would. I placed those items as the top five on my list. The positive consequences were a little easier to list once I had researched the negative consequences." Jason paused and then remarked, "I'm actually pretty proud of my lists."

"Good to hear," David said, beaming. "I'm proud of you for keeping your commitment to follow the program. I'm eager to go over it with you. But before we go over the lists, tell me a little more about your research process. Did you find most of the items on your list from reading academic research?"

"The academic research was interesting, and it laid out some serious negative consequences from rigorous studies. But the real-life stories hit home with me even more. I found that the consequences on both lists were similar."

"Show me your list," David requested.

Jason smiled at David's eagerness to look at the lists. He felt the satisfaction of accomplishment and the warmth of approval. Jason opened the binder that he used for his discussions with David to the following list.

Top Five Negative Consequences of Viewing and Doing:

1. **Decreased capacity to love. Increased anger toward spouse and children. Difficulties in relationships with others and God.**
2. **Marital disharmony. Lack of sexual intimacy. Poor regard for spouse.**
3. **Self-loathing, lack of self-esteem and confidence.**
4. **Guilt, fear, and depression and numbed emotions.**
5. **Poor performance at work.**

"It looks like you may have compiled a list of fifteen to twenty items but grouped them to narrow it to five," David said, laughing.

"I know it looks that way, but let me explain. The first consequence that struck me as being true in my case and harmful not just to me but also to my family is the decreased capacity to love. The research, stories, and reactions I read that came from spouses and children all pointed to this as a major consequence.

"I believe the increased anger toward those we love most—or should love most—and the difficulties in relationships are a result of the decreased capacity to love. I also think that viewing pornography is repugnant in the Creator's sight, so one loses His light when he or she views. I believe He is the source of love, so it's natural that love would decrease when one is engaged in a viewing habit.

"This rang true with my religious beliefs and was confirmed by the academic studies. I was a little surprised."

"What caused the surprise?"

"In the past, I often thought that nothing was really wrong with viewing pornography, except that my parents and church taught me that it was wrong. Growing up with those beliefs made me feel guilty for viewing. I thought that if could overcome the guilt from growing up in a prudish household, I would be normal and fine.

"Based upon the research, the personal experiences I read, and how they both ring true to my own experience, I now believe that the loss of the capacity to love is a natural consequence for everyone who views. It is not just a product of a socially conservative upbringing. All of the evidence I found, including academic research, points to the fact that a viewer loses some—I personally think it's a lot—of his or her ability to love others."

David listened intently. Jason was encouraged by David's attentiveness and continued. "What do you think?"

David paused before answering, searching his memory. "I can't think of a viewer I'm aware of who didn't suffer from a lower capacity to love and to feel love. Based upon those I've counseled, I like to use the description that viewers' capacity to love drops like a rock. Viewers rarely see their limited capacity to love until they have a lengthy period of true abstinence and see some of that capacity restored.

"A lot of the academic research you referred to that relates to this consequence discusses the bonding that takes place between pornographic images and the viewer. This bonding prevents bonding between spouse, potential spouse, family members, or others and the viewer.

David continued, "I don't normally like to make judgments on someone's personal consequences list, but I think this is one of the biggest negative consequences of viewing and doing, so I'm glad you listed it first. Please continue."

"I guess you could tie number two, marital disharmony, lack of sexual intimacy, and poor regard for one's spouse, back to number one, but I thought it was so important that it should stand on its own. I haven't felt deep love for my wife in years, and to me, it clearly ties back to my pornography use.

"I mean, it is clear now that my pornography use harms my ability to love my wife. It wasn't so clear to me before the research. I thought that she was at least partly to blame."

Jason continued, speaking quickly. "My ability to connect with her physically is also harmed. The pleasure I receive from pornography is robbing me of the joy I could have from sexual intimacy with my wife. My alienation from her and my viewing her as another object pushes us further apart. I didn't even realize until I was doing this homework that I viewed her as an object and a means to my sexual satisfaction.

"I often secretly blame her for my addiction, thinking that if she were willing to have sex more often, I wouldn't turn to pornography. I realize now that this is a lie, and I'm the one causing marital disharmony."

David interrupted Jason at this point. "I'm glad you acknowledged you may be to blame. That is a key component of healing, and we'll get into it in more detail later when we discuss increasing personal responsibility and getting rid of victim language."

"I've learned that when someone has a viewing habit, he or she can't love his or her spouse deeply. This exercise helped me realize that my addiction is the problem in our marriage; the problem isn't anything that she is doing.

"As I was researching, I also thought about how I've recently felt somewhat out of love with Becky. Her faults seem big, and she isn't as pretty to me as she used to be. I then recalled my porn-free, or life of love time. During those months, I felt more in love with her and saw more of her good qualities than her faults; I noticed how good-looking she really is to me.

"I had the strong impression that it was my viewing and doing that caused me to feel out of love, magnify her faults, and forget how beautiful she was to me. It was a powerful experience."

David observed, "I'm impressed with the depth of your feelings about the first two consequences. Do you see the value in compiling the list yourself? I could have provided you with one, but you wouldn't have internalized the consequences to the same degree. And your understanding of your personal experience would not have been enhanced like it was."

Jason was eager to continue telling David about his experience. "I think you're right. Let me tell you more about number three and the feelings I've had." Jason was excited about his discovery of consequences that had been cloudy for a long time.

"Number three, the self-loathing and lack of confidence, came from some of the academic studies I found on the Internet that were from a religious angle. Professors who were also men and women of faith had performed research on the effects of pornography. They described an increase in self-hatred, an increase in depression, and a drop in self-confidence as natural consequences of pornography that impact the entire life of the addict.

"This rang true to me. I often ascribed these feelings to my conservative religious upbringing, but now I believe that they are natural, real consequences of viewing and doing. I deeply experience self-hatred and diminished self-confidence. I don't feel like I will amount to much if I can't control this addiction. I also don't feel bold enough to take on projects, initiatives, community service, or some of the activities I used to do.

"The cloudiness surrounding the lack of confidence is going away as I see the low opinion I have of myself and how it makes me quick to get angry and blame others; it also makes me impatient and slow to forgive. I can see more clearly the impact viewing has on my interaction with others—especially my family but even my colleagues."

Jason looked down at the floor for a moment and then continued.

"I'm sorry if what I included in number four—guilt, fear, depression, and numb emotions—seems similar to number three, but to me, they were distinct consequences. Maybe the guilt, shame, and depression lead to self-loathing, lack of self-esteem, and lack of self-confidence. The feelings are strong, so I wanted to list them separately."

David nodded in approval of Jason's list.

"Sometimes the depression and feeling of being trapped or the guilt and shame from stooping to something I know is wrong can be overwhelming. I feel like I'm doing something wrong, and I know it, but I can't stop.

"I used to vow after every incident that it was the last, and my guilt, shame, and depression increased every time I broke that vow. More recently, I didn't think I could keep the promise to myself, so I stopped making it. But the shame and guilt don't go away, and the depression is real.

"I think the absence of spirituality in my life leaves a void filled with guilt, shame, and depression. I also think my inability to leave something alone when I know it's bad creates a lot of guilt and self-doubt. That's why I was so concerned about failing if this program required me to use self-discipline—I don't have any.

"I used to think that the guilt and shame I felt originated from my religious upbringing, but I saw them both discussed as consequences in the academic studies. I believe it's morally wrong to view and do, but even if I didn't, the guilt and shame would still be there. The simple fact that I can't stop doing it produces guilt and shame. I guess the addiction leads me to believe that I'm less of a person that I thought I was.

"Number five, 'poor performance at work,' was something I had partially realized before doing the research, but it really hit home as I studied and pondered it. I used to feel like I could separate the pornography addiction from my work life, but the stories I read made me feel that poor performance at work is a natural consequence of viewing and doing. It probably has to do with the decreased ability to have meaningful relationships and the lack of self-confidence.

"It may also have something to do with the amount of time I spend viewing and doing that others are spending focused on sharpening their skills or actually performing work. Regardless, I believe my progress at the office has been stalled by my pornography habit."

Jason paused. He was breathing heavily after talking passionately. David smiled. "What a great list, Jason. I think your research paid off. I doubt that any of these consequences felt new to you. You had probably subtly realized that they were natural consequences of your addiction, but now you have clarified them. To go back to our analogies, you cleared the clouds, and now the consequences are clearer.

"Before we move on to the list of positive consequences in living life without pornography, could you share with me some of the consequences you excluded from your list?"

Jason showed David his lengthy list of other negative consequences. As David glanced at the list, Jason commented, "I could have spent several more hours compiling the list of negative consequences to choose from. I decided I had enough, so I turned my focus to the positive list."

David looked up. "Yes, you have quite a list. I'm glad you included some of the serious consequences on your list. I'm impressed that you included many references as well so you can reread the context in the future. Referring to this list regularly is an important part of keeping the clouds away." David continued reading the list.

Negative Consequences:

Severe consequences due to sexual behavior and an inability to stop despite these adverse consequences. In Patrick Carnes's book, *Don't Call It Love*, 1991, some of the losses reported by sex addicts include:

Loss of partner or spouse (40 percent)
Severe marital or relationship problems (70 percent)
Loss of career opportunities (27 percent)
Unwanted pregnancies (40 percent)
Abortions (36 percent)
Suicide obsession (72 percent)
Suicide attempts (17 percent)
Exposure to AIDS and venereal disease (68 percent)
Legal risks from nuisance offenses to rape (58 percent)

Dramatically reduced capacity to love.

Marked dissociation of sex from friendship, affection, caring, and other normal healthy emotions and traits that help marital and family relationships. Victor B. Cline, *Treatment and Healing of Pornographic and Sexual Addictions,* April 1999.

Repeatedly masturbating to deviant pornographic imagery (either as memories or with explicit external pornographic stimuli risks (via conditioning) the acquiring of sexual addictions and other sexual pathology. Cline, *Treatment and Healing of Pornographic and Sexual Addictions.*

"Marital or couple disharmony, sometimes divorce, and sometimes the breaking up of other valued relationships." Cline, *Treatment and Healing of Pornographic and Sexual Addictions.*

Loss of free agency. Cline, *Treatment and Healing of Pornographic and Sexual Addictions.*

Strong correlation between pornography and sex crimes. Stan Weed, "Pornography: a review of scientific literature," *National Coalition for the Protection of Children and Families.*

Miss a profound opportunity for what many have described as a spiritual connection between ourselves, our spouse, and God, in exchange for the temporary gratification of our individual lusts and desires. Jeffrey R. Holland, "Personal Purity," *Ensign,* November 1998.

Difficulties in their relationship with themselves, with others, and with God. Being thus cut off from these sources of emotional strength, the person is then more susceptible to the influence of negative thoughts and beliefs that end up in their minds. Jeffrey R. Holland, "Personal Purity."

Destructive emotional avoidance strategies. Jason Briere, "Trauma: assessment and treatment in adult interpersonal violence" (Presentation given at annual Treatment Conference of the Utah Domestic Advisory Council, 2000).

Development of compulsive behavior patterns as we find that pornography use temporarily relieves our negative feelings. Paul James Birch *Pornography Use: Consequences and Cures.*

Negative feelings (guilt, shame, etc.) A. Dean Byrd and Mark Chamberlain, *Willpower is not enough: Why we don't succeed at change,* Deseret Book, 1995, Ch. 1, and Carnes, Out of the shadows, pp. 99–116.

More susceptible to problems in relationships because there is a sense of feeling cut off or isolated in their shame. Birch, *Pornography Use: Consequences and Cures.*

Depression, low self-worth, hopelessness, fear, guilt, shame, financial problems, eating problems, anxiety disorders, inability to deal with sexual abuse issues, inability to form lasting relationships, idealization of hoped for relationships, intense criticism of actual relationships, disturbances in relationships (particularly spousal and parental). Birch, *Pornography Use: Consequences and Cures.*

Progress is washed away with each relapse. Birch, *Pornography Use: Consequences and Cures.*

Marital happiness, self-esteem, stress management, parenting relationships, etc., are all potentially compromised. Birch, *Pornography Use: Consequences and Cures.*

Decreased sexual desire for spouse. Bridges, A.J., Bergner, R.M., "Romantic partners' use of pornography: Its significance for women," *Journal of Sex and Marital Therapy,* 29, 1–14.

Decreased sexual intimacy. Schneider, J.P. (1998). "The new "elephant in the living room:" Effects of compulsive cybersex behaviors on the spouse." *CyberPsychology and Behavior,* 1(2), 169–186.

It will destroy your home life. It will destroy your marriage. It will take the good and beautiful out of your family relationships and replace these with ugliness and suspicion. Gordon B Hinckley, *Ensign,* November 2000.

Overspending and Debt. Manning, J.C. (2005). *A qualitative study of the supports women find most beneficial when dealing with a spouse's sexually addictive or compulsive sexual behavior.* Doctoral Dissertation.

"Social life suffered. So did my schoolwork, family ties, and—most important—my spirituality." "Danger Ahead! Avoiding Pornography's Trap," *New Era,* Oct 2002, p. 34.

"At the very time I most needed the promptings of the Spirit in my life, I was less and less able to feel anything. Life became a constant struggle against depression." "Danger Ahead! Avoiding Pornography's Trap," *New Era*.

"My soul hungered, but the only thing I fed it offered no nourishment. I would get down on myself, so I would delve into pornography to feel better. But the pornography would upset me even more." "Danger Ahead! Avoiding Pornography's Trap" *New Era*.

"Guilt, fear, and depression are common emotions for those involved with pornography—guilt, because they know what they are doing is wrong; fear, because they are terrified their secret will be found out; and depression, because they no longer feel the Spirit." Breaking the Chains of Pornography, Ensign, Feb 2001.

Relationships with family, friends, church leaders, and the Lord are damaged. Breaking the Chains of Pornography, Ensign, Feb 2001.

"My self-confidence dwindled in church, school, and everywhere. Many times I felt very alone, awkward, and unworthy. If a girl liked me, I would think, 'She wouldn't like me if she *really* knew me.' I would shy away from being social." Breaking the Chains of Pornography, *Ensign*, Feb 2001.

"I noticed a change in my own countenance day by day, year by year. I became calloused and hardened. I found myself lying to my parents, my bishop, everyone around me. Inside I was going through personal turmoil and spiritual torment." Breaking the Chains of Pornography, *Ensign*, Feb 2001.

"I loathed myself." Breaking the Chains of Pornography, *Ensign*, Feb 2001.

"Numbs the feelings." Breaking the Chains of Pornography, *Ensign*, Feb 2001.

There were a few more items on the list, but David's face showed some strain. He recognized the cold feeling that came with reading so many negative consequences, including those that devastate the lives of a viewer and his or her family. He put the list down and stated, "That's enough of the negative. Show me your positive consequences list. We will build on that as our main goal today."

Jason turned the page in his binder and showed the list to David.

Top Five Positive Consequences of Living a Loving Life:

1. **Increased love for spouse, kids, and others I care about, leading to deeper relationships.**
2. **Marital harmony. Greater regard and deeper love for spouse. Rekindled spark.**
3. **Strong performance at work.**
4. **Happiness. Spiritual connection. More depth of emotions.**
5. **Self-confidence, self-love. Getting my swagger back.**

David smiled. "This looks a lot like the list of negatives."

"I guess the positive consequences that are the most important to me are the opposite of the negative consequences I most fear."

Jason looked at David, waiting for a reaction. The concerned look on David's face puzzled Jason.

David started speaking slowly. "I'm worried that you may have, not deliberately, taken a shortcut with the process for this list."

Jason was still puzzled. "What do you mean?"

"What I really liked about your negative consequences list was the passion and the personal discoveries you made during the research process. You owned the negative consequences. You believed they applied to you in a personal and real manner.

"I feel confident that you've begun the process to keep the negative consequences cloud-free because you believe them deeply and personally. I don't feel the same passion about the personal discoveries and ownership of the positive consequences. Can you help me understand why?

"I've found over the years that the men and women who succeed in overcoming viewing and doing are the ones who do it for themselves.

"I've had several people come see me for the same training you're here to experience. Some come because they're tired of living with viewing and happen to meet someone who is familiar with our program. Some people are here after trying other programs and failing. Some show up because their spouse discovered their behavior and demanded they get help. Others come because a therapist convinced them it was necessary for their marriage. And some are here under a court order for help with deeper sexual addictions.

"I've found that regardless of why someone initially comes to us, those who identify the negative and positive consequences that matter most to them—not to their families, their therapists, or their judge—are the ones who succeed. Because they feel a personal connection and belief in the negative and positive consequences, they are more likely to succeed than those whose attitude is that they are doing it for someone else rather than themselves.

"I want to help you assess whether the items on your positive consequences list capture the passion and personal ownership to keep the clouds at bay and take the power back from viewing. Does that make sense?"

Jason thought for a moment and then said, "I think my passion and ownership is solid, but I didn't follow your directions precisely, so that may be reflected in my lists. I researched the larger list of both negative and positive consequences before picking my top five of each. I think that if I would have talked about the positive consequences first, you would have felt the same passion and detail as I showed for the negatives list.

"Because I refined the larger lists of negatives and positives down to five at the same time, the lists look similar. But some of the after parts of the before-and-after experiences from others who've overcome viewing struck me as very positive, and I felt ownership, belief, and a strong desire to experience the positive consequences myself."

The smile returned to David's face. "Great. Thanks for that explanation. I'm sorry I took us off track briefly, but now you know how important this part of the program is.

"I want to pause now and talk a little bit about the phrases we use to refer to not viewing. When we state our goal as 'not viewing pornography,' we are expressing a desire to refrain from an action with negative consequences. However, when we state our goal as 'living a loving life,' we express a desire to take action that provides positive consequences."

"I'm not sure what the difference is. What do you mean?" Jason asked.

"You'll find out in the next session how important it is to focus on the positive consequences of living a loving life, so don't worry, you'll see the difference clearly at that point. But before we go on, could you go over the positive consequences with me? I liked your summary of the negatives and would love to hear the same thing with the positives."

Jason was still animated. "Of course. When I think about number one, increased love for those most important to me, it became crystal clear that not only was this a natural consequence of not view—oops, I mean of living a life of love—but also how vitally important a deep, loving relationship with my wife is to my happiness.

"It seemed like everything I read pointed to these relationships being the key to happiness in life. I don't mean to sound surprised; I've known deep down that it's true. It's just that it had been a little cloudy for me until doing this research."

David smiled at Jason's use of the word "cloudy." He was getting it.

"This increased love is not only a positive benefit but also a high-priority goal so that I can really live my life with those I love. I don't want to just coast through life, tolerating people but feeling anger and hatred toward them because of my viewing and doing addiction. I truly believe that the relationships I develop and maintain with my wife, kids, and other family members as well as friends are vital to my happiness and well-being.

"Number two, better marriage relationship and better regard for my wife, is similar to number one, but I think it better captures how living a loving life can help me respect her and not objectify her. Instead of expecting her to act like a porn star, this will help me love her for who she is.

"It was interesting to see that unmarried men and women of all ages encountered the same benefit with the women and men in their lives. They had a much easier time building and maintaining connections with those they dated or wanted to date. They saw and respected the person as he or she really is and not as an object. They were also able to determine with much greater certainty if the person was marriage-worthy because they were seeing him or her through non-viewer eyes.

"I was fascinated by the experiences singles shared about the question of marriage-worthiness. It was clear that the blindness caused by viewing hurt their ability to see beyond the sexual relationship, or potential sexual relationship, to evaluating the things they had in common, their compatibility, and their ability to be best friends in marriage. If I were single, this would probably be the biggest consequence for me. Who you marry is such an important decision, and to have it clouded over by the effects of viewing would make a wise decision almost impossible.

"We touched on number three, strong performance at work, when we covered the negative consequences, but I was a little surprised at how clear this benefit was in all the personal stories I read. Improved work or school performance always followed recovery. I thought about the ways I could advance in my company or join another company at a higher level.

"For adolescents, the pickup in school grades was clear: students' grades improved generally but clearly when they started living a loving life. I say 'generally' because some studies showed that student viewers were able to maintain high grades, but their learning was inferior to students living a loving life. I researched the consequences to adolescents because that's when I started viewing."

David nodded his head. Jason could tell that the benefits were not new to David, but he was enjoying hearing Jason's personal insights into them.

"Number four, increased happiness, greater spiritual connection, and greater depth of emotions, was very present in the research, both academic and religious. I don't think anyone can maintain a spiritual connection, no matter how they define it, when viewing or doing. There is too much natural shame and guilt. But the feelings of freedom, general happiness, spiritual connection, and an ability to see and appreciate beauty when men went from being viewers to living a loving life were clear.

"I could spend more time on this one because it's such a huge positive consequence and it really rang true to me, but I think you get the picture." David nodded his approval.

"I think number five, increased self-confidence, goes along with the rest. When someone can love others and feel deeply, that person can have self-confidence. But it's also deeper than that. When you live a loving life, you feel more in control of yourself, your time, and your life in general. The feeling of control, especially some control over viewing, gives you confidence. I found that self-confidence was also a natural result of living a loving life."

"Thanks, Jason. I can tell that researching the consequences was a great experience for you. I would guess that you spent a lot of time on your homework."

"Yeah. I probably spent over four hours, but it zoomed by and only felt like one."

"I hope you see the value of clarifying consequences that have become cloudy with time and with our rationalizations."

Jason smiled as he said, "I can't think of a more valuable use of the four hours. It was a profound experience for me, and it truly lifted the clouds on consequences that I knew were there. It also made me aware of consequences I had not yet associated with viewing and doing. Thanks for giving me the homework."

"If you will review your top five lists of negative and positive consequences regularly, you'll gain strength to live a loving life and overcome the power of the lustful thoughts and feelings that viewing produces."

In response to the doubt in Jason's face, David added, "You're probably wondering, especially now that the consequences are so clear in your mind, why you need to review them regularly." Jason was getting used to David knowing what he was thinking, so he just nodded.

"Our minds like to focus on the immediate consequences and forget about the long-term ones. If we don't review all of them regularly, they become cloudy again and drift further from our minds. When this happens, we over-emphasize immediate gratification, start viewing again, and then become subject to the negative consequences.

"In terms of our brain, if we don't interrupt the stimulus-response of the reptilian brain by bringing the logical brain to the forefront, our brain reverts back to its old wiring, responding to the stimulus or trigger and focusing on satisfying it by viewing and doing. Does this make sense?"

As soon as David asked this, Jason felt that it was true in his own life.

David continued, "We'll discuss the power of repetition in detail later, but I want to mention it now because of how it applies to this step. Sometimes repetition gets a bad name. We associate it with being boring and mindless or with requiring little expansion of ourselves. However, repetition is a powerful force in realizing goals and developing positive habits.

"When you repeat a goal frequently in writing and in speaking, it becomes part of you. Achieving it then becomes almost inevitable. In essence, you take something that typically stays in the vague recesses of your mind and bring it to the forefront.

"The same applies to repeating the consequences, both negative and positive, with more emphasis on the positive. When you repeat them regularly, they move to the forefront, and you reflect them in your actions naturally and with greater ease.

"When you neglect reviewing or repeating them for a while, they become cloudy, seeking to return to the vague recesses of your mind. Then, in moments of challenge, they do not readily come forth to aid you.

"Does this make sense?"

As Jason thought about the way his mind worked, he nodded his head in agreement.

"Another way to put it is that the repetition helps rewire a new pathway in our brain, but the old pathway remains. As we continue to practice the new action, the new pathway gets increasingly bright, and the old pathway grows dimmer. But if we stop practicing, the new pathway grows dim, and the likelihood increases that we revive the old pathway of viewing and doing.

"You've probably heard at work that 'defining the problem is fifty percent of the solution.' In this case, defining and clarifying the consequences may be half of the solution to overcoming your pornography addiction.

"To gain greater power over pornography, you'll need the other fifty percent. Are you ready to move to step two in our next session?"

Jason understood this, so he nodded to let David know he was ready to move to the next step.

"Before we move on, I have one point to reiterate about clarifying consequences. It's important for you to focus particularly on the positive consequences of living a loving life. That's why we do them after the negative ones. When you review your consequences, you'll benefit much more from the positive ones; the clearer and more emotion-filled these are to you, the better.

"To keep the clouds away and to continue to start forming a new neural pathway, your homework this session is about repetition."

Homework for the Negative and Positive Consequences:

1. Rank your top five negative and positive consequences and list them in priority order, from the most meaningful and impactful to the least.

2. Rewrite your reordered negative and positive consequences list (keep the clouds away with repetition) once per day while reciting them, aloud if possible.
3. Reread the key concepts from this lesson.

Note: *Please refer to* poweroverpornography.com/consequences *for the latest additions to the negative consequences of pornography and for the positive consequences of living a loving life. Please feel welcome to contribute additional consequences that you've experienced or discovered in your research.*

CHAPTER 6:

The Power of Vision

Vivid Vision

David wrote on the whiteboard, "'Where there is no vision, the people perish' (Prov. 29:18)."

"The second—and possibly the most important—step in your training is developing your vision, specifically relating to overcoming your addiction. You'll come to see how the power of your vision can lift you above your addiction.

"You already suggested that you are at risk of losing the love of your family if you persist in viewing and doing. Based upon your discussion of positive consequences at our last session, I believe that you, like me, consider your relationships with your family to be one of the most worthwhile parts of life. Using the terminology of the verse from Proverbs, I think we can relate losing the love of our family to perishing. It's not quite the same, but they are similar feelings. Life's richness is diminished greatly without our family relationships.

"I think you'll find it interesting that even for teens, the most worthwhile relationships are with their families. Teens suffering from a viewing and doing addiction tend to take their anger out on their parents and siblings, so they lose that love when viewing. But they get it back strongly when they live a loving life. Just ask their parents." David smiled.

Jason didn't smile back. "Jason, you seem a little fidgety. Is something on your mind?"

"I had a great experience with clarifying consequences and keeping the clouds away from them, but I'm not feeling it with the vision thing. It seems a little out there to me. I guess my cynical self is starting to creep into my thoughts."

"I'm glad you let me know how you're feeling. Let me describe it this way: you'll develop a simple, two or three-sentence vision statement that builds on the list of positive consequences.

"The vision statement you develop will be a powerful driver in your overcoming viewing and doing. You may have to extend your trust a little more, but it all comes together within a few sessions, and you'll see how a strong vision will provide you with power when you are tempted to view. Do you think you can relax and do that?"

"Sure. Based upon the power I felt from making the consequences list, I feel like this is headed in the right direction."

"Great. Let's continue. Before we can create a new reality for ourselves, we have to be able to create it in a vision. Consider the words of James Allen, author of the essay 'As a Man Thinketh.'"

He who cherishes a beautiful vision, a lofty ideal in his heart, will one day realize it. Columbus cherished a vision of another world, and he discovered it; Copernicus fostered a vision of a multiplicity of worlds and a wider universe, and he revealed it; Buddha beheld the vision of a spiritual world of stainless beauty and perfect peace, and he entered into it.

"Our next step in gaining power over pornography is to create your positive vision of living a loving life. I want to reiterate the importance of phrasing overcoming pornography in a positive way.

"Before we move to the positive consequences of living a loving life, let's talk about the power of positive.

"When you are reaching for positive goals and consequences, you will be motivated to take the action necessary to achieve them. When you are focused on avoiding negative consequences, you will tend to feel demotivated and to be filled with fear and anxiety. We'll spend some time creating a vision out of your positive consequences within the next few modules.

"By the way, positive consequences that relate to others and not directly to you aren't typically inspiring enough. In the future, we'll talk about how the consequences need to focus on you directly.

"You know about many of the negative consequences, yet you've persisted in viewing and doing. Therefore, clearly the negative consequences alone do not have the power to stop a viewing and doing habit.

"Let me illustrate how focusing on the negative is usually not the way to the solution. Please look out the window but don't imagine a purple hippopotamus standing on your car, crushing the roof and hood."

Jason understood immediately. "I get it. I pictured a cartoon-like animated hippopotamus smiling as he smashed my car. I couldn't get the image out of my mind."

"So if your vision focuses on not thinking about pornography, what word will you not be able to get out of your mind?"

"Pornography."

"Precisely. If you phrase your desire to overcome pornography as 'not viewing pornography,' the word left in your mind is 'pornography.' Therefore, you'll want to infuse your vision with positive statements and words, not with overcoming negative statements. In other words: your mind will want to focus on the picture you give it, so give it a positive picture.

"If you're ever tempted to state your vision or other goals in terms of avoiding the negative, correct yourself by thinking of the purple hippo. If you're focusing on getting him off your car, he'll stay around, stomping dent marks all over it.

"I think you'll like the vision development process, but it requires more homework. This homework is vital to the development of a vivid, positive vision for yourself. In turn, the vision is vital to your recovery.

"Speaking of homework, one reason I asked you to rank and rewrite your positive consequences list was to make sure you keep the consequences at the top of your mind so they can form the foundation for your vision. We'll get back to that in a minute, but let's establish the foundation first.

"Before we launch into developing your vision, I want to emphasize its power to you. I think that addictions, including viewing and doing addictions, keep many people from achieving their dreams. However, being addiction-free isn't the only requirement for achieving one's dreams. While addicts and the unambitious view life as unfair and themselves as victims, those who develop and then pursue a passionate vision find that life and achievement work out for them.

"In fact, your vision determines more than anything else your future. More important than the way you were raised, your individual circumstances or who your parents were, your personal vision will determine your realized potential.

"Why is vision so important? It reflects the best life you want to live. All visions encounter opposition but powerful visions have the power to overcome all obstacles and can drive you past the most powerful opposition or setback.

"What is the difference between the vision with enough power to overcome all obstacles and the one that doesn't? The empowering vision has the following three attributes: One, it needs to be well-defined. A blurry vision doesn't have pulling power. Two, it needs to be vivid. A black and white vision won't help you power through obstacles like a vivid, colorful, clear vision will. In fact, the more tangible your vision, the more power you have. Three, it needs to be positive. Focusing on the negative never seems to work.

"I recently hiked a few hours on a trail in the Rocky Mountains that early pioneers in the Western United States blazed over 160 years ago. The section I hiked was the longest uphill portion of the entire journey. Although not the steepest incline, the incline didn't let up for the entire section. While I was able to hike this portion of the trail in a few hours, the early pioneers took over one week, having to cut through a lot of brush and timber along the way and carry all of their earthly belongings with them in wagons or handcarts.

"As I thought about how hard that must have been, I thought, 'What gave them the strength to continue each day with insufficient food, clothing, shoes and provisions?' I believe it was their vision. Every day they saw in their minds the new life that they would live in a new land with untold promise for them and their families. I'll bet they saw themselves in their new homes surrounded with loved ones.

"How else could they power themselves up and over the many obstacles they faced almost every day? Despite witnessing the death of friends and family along the way and suffering from extreme weather, their vision gave them power to get up and push through whatever they faced.

"When modern pioneers encounter obstacles, resistance and opposition, those with powerful visions power through them, many times while not even thinking about the opposition. They focus on the finish of the race while running it and focus on the outcome and associated celebration when fully engaged in a huge endeavor. They are willing to do hard, uncomfortable tasks to make their visions come to pass.

"Jason, when you think about the most important concepts of vision, what comes to mind?"

Jason paused, considering what David had just said as well as his own thoughts on vision. "Quite a few thoughts come to mind:

"Nothing has as much power for affecting your future as your ability to have a vision.

Vision is a projection of the kind of life you want to live.

Vision can drive you to great achievement.

Vision sets in motion forces that can overpower any obstacle in your path.

A powerful vision is well-defined. A blurry vision has little pulling power.

To really have your vision pull you forward, it must be vivid and nearly tangible.

High achievers' vision is focused on the positive, not the resistance.

High achievers' vision is stronger than the obstacles they face.

To achieve your vision, you need to be willing to do hard and uncomfortable tasks."

"Thanks. Now, let's focus on the attributes of vision that make it powerful and enable it to drive achievement. What attributes from our discussion or your experience make a vision powerful enough to drive action?"

"I don't have much experience with vision, but a few things stood out from our discussion. The phrases 'well-defined,' 'vivid,' and 'focus on the positive' are the ones that were notable."

"Those struck me as well. Let's start crafting a vision for you that is well-defined, vivid, and positive. If your mind can see your vision clearly, it will be better able to maintain it as a force to drive achievement. And for your mind to see it clearly, your vision needs to be well-defined, vivid, and positive."

David turned to the whiteboard to write the last statement.

"Jason, would you retrieve your notebook and review your newly ranked five positive consequences of living a loving life? Both the review and the homework will help you form the basis of your vision."

Jason pulled his notebook from his briefcase as he started talking. "I thought this homework assignment was going to be much easier than the last one, but I struggled to rank the positive consequences. I reviewed them all and decided that the first priority is increased love for my wife and kids. I really want more love in my relationships."

Jason handed the notebook to David and added, "You can see how I reordered the other consequences. Although performing well at work is important to me and my self-image, regaining my self-confidence and reconnecting spiritually are more important to me."

David read through the list:

1. Increased love for spouse, kids, and others I care about leading to deeper, more meaningful relationships.
2. Marital harmony. Greater regard and deeper love for spouse. Rekindled spark.

3. Self-confidence, self-love. Get my swagger back.
4. Happiness. Spiritual connection. More depth of emotions.
5. Stronger performance at work.

David said, "I think that is an excellent number one, and I'm glad you put the thought into ranking the others. Your goal now will be to review the list of ranked positive consequences and begin to formulate a vivid vision.

"As you look through the positives, are there any themes that stand out that can be components of your vision? Remember, your vision is what you want your life to be as a result of living a loving life."

As Jason looked at the list, four things that he strongly desired to be part of his future life stood out to him.

"Love, personal, marital, and family happiness, self-confidence, and work achievement stand out as important parts. Maybe we can start with those."

"OK. I think these can be part of your vision, but let's try to make them more vivid so that your mind can picture them easily. First, increased love is a definite result from living a loving life. The first quality that declines when a person views pornography is his or her capability to love. The difference can seem subtle to the viewer, but it's generally stark to family members. This change often results in the viewer's expression of anger, perhaps through a shorter temper, and in his or her magnification of others' flaws.

"I believe love should be part of every viewer's vision statement because it is so vital to developing and maintaining strong relationships, and it is such an important component of happiness. Tell me how you can make love a clear, vivid part of your vision."

"That's a little like the high school English assignment to describe love or other emotions. I struggled in coming up with a concrete definition."

"Think about the ideal loving relationship with your wife and kids. Maybe it would help to think of a scene in the future that you could experience as a result of living a loving life."

Jason started sharing his thoughts. "Your statement about magnifying flaws is sticking in my mind. I've been focusing on my wife's weaknesses and thinking that my kids need discipline to correct all the things they do wrong.

"As I think about it, I'm pretty sure their wrongs and weaknesses are ordinary, but I'm blowing them out of proportion. I've come to believe that my perspective is a consequence of my viewing and doing."

He replayed the scene of his arrival home just two nights ago and how he had blamed his wife and children for a miserable evening. As Jason thought about David's words, he realized that the miserable evening was his own fault. His lack of love for his family, caused by his viewing, was truly destroying his most important relationships.

David sensed that Jason was still stuck in the negative past. "Jason, sometimes putting yourself in a certain happy place within your vision can help you get started."

Jason smiled at the phrase "happy place." He thought of the fun that he had as a kid at the lake, fishing and boating with his family. He had written in his journal as a boy that the lake was a happy place. He continued to enjoy it as an adult. He knew his wife enjoyed it as well, more for the beauty than the fishing and boating, although she seemed to like waterskiing.

"How about this? I envision feeling deep mutual love and togetherness with my wife and children as we watch the sun set over the lake."

"Great start. What else from your positive consequences list do you want to capture in your vision?"

"I want to capture it all, but if it's too long, it will lose some of its realness. I think I would like to capture the self-confidence and better performance at work. How does this sound? 'Boldly advance in the office with outstanding performance.'"

David didn't seem to like this part as much. "You're definitely right about not wanting to make it too long. Soon, you will review your vision in your mind frequently, so you'll want to make sure it follows the KIS principle."

Jason thought of the statement, "Keep it simple, stupid." He preferred the added *S* on the end to emphasize the message. They referred frequently to the KIS(S) principle often at his job.

David continued, "Is the career performance part of your vision vivid enough to evoke emotion? Emotion has more power to drive our behavior and actions than intellect does."

Jason thought for a few seconds, and then he suggested, "Feel deep love for my wife and children as we watch the sun set over the lake and I watch their smiles. Feel confident and satisfied, knowing that my excellent performance on the job drives success there."

"Great progress. I sense more emotion in this version. I also get some of the vividness from your mention of the sunset, the lake, and smiles. The phrase 'deep love' has emotion but isn't quite so vivid. Same with 'confident' and 'satisfied.' Any thoughts on how to make them a bit more alive, a bit more tangible, so you can picture them vividly?"

"I'm drawing a blank."

"That's OK. Sometimes our minds need time to simmer on a thought before they come up with the right solution. Why don't you let this one do that for a bit and then focus on it later today or tomorrow to make it more vivid?"

Jason wasn't ready to wait. Before David could move on, he blurted out, "How about this? 'I will demonstrate my deep love for my wife and kids by hugging, laughing, listening, talking, and spending time doing what they like to do, accompanied by smiles and sunsets at the lake. I'll confidently complete top-notch work on time, exceeding expectations and feeling that I deserve the promotion.'"

"Winner, winner, chicken dinner."

Jason couldn't hold back his laughter. He didn't expect to hear this expression from an old guy like David.

David smiled and chuckled at Jason's reaction. "It sounds like that vision is vivid for you." They both laughed.

David captured some of the important components of vision on the whiteboard:

"I like your vision statement, but here are a couple suggestions. It's important that your benefits be for you. Your family will naturally benefit, but they should be secondary beneficiaries. This will give you a higher chance of success. You currently have three different visions that will be hard to keep clear: hugs, sunsets, and top-notch work. Brevity is important in defining your vision because it will be something you refer to over and over. You want it to roll off your tongue easily and paint the same picture in your mind every time. You also want it to be simple."

"Hmm. I like what you're saying. What if I change it to: 'Show my deep love for my wife and kids by hugging, laughing, listening, talking, and spending time doing what we like and confidently initiating and completing work that exceeds expectations'?

"I hate to lose the lake and sunsets, but I don't think they tied in quite so well as the other components. Now I'm down to two. Do you think it's OK?"

"Great improvements. I think it meets the criteria, but the important question is, do you?" David wrote on the whiteboard as he asked the following questions of Jason: "Does it paint a picture in your mind? Are the benefits directly yours, not others? Is it brief? Is it easy to say? Is it simple?"

The accountant in Jason came out. "Hey, it's the rule of five again. Let me see if it meets them." Jason began thinking out loud again.

"It paints a clear picture in my mind of me with my wife and with my kids, hugging and laughing together. I can imagine my sense of humor coming back. I've changed the benefits to be more for me than for my family. It's not the briefest, but I think I can keep it in my mind. It's not too hard to say, but I can work on that part. I think it's pretty simple.

"So far, I think it does meet the criteria, but I'll let it simmer for a while and come back to it to make any changes."

"Well, I think that's enough for today. I hope you're starting to sense that this is different than what you've tried before, and it has some power to help you. I think you'll discover effective principles in the upcoming sessions when we talk about the power of acknowledging and accepting and the power to choose. In fact, there is power in these simple concepts that you never thought possible. You'll also learn why your power to choose is crucial to the program.

"Don't forget the homework. Your vision is merely a wish if you don't continue vivifying it, making it sufficiently brief, and repeating it so that it becomes a part of you."

David drove home feeling a little lighter. Instead of listening to the market report like he often would have done, he listened to his favorite music station and sang along with the music all the way home.

Homework for Vision:

1. Write your five ranked positive benefits of living a loving life. Repeat them in your mind three times each.
2. Write your vision statement five times. Remove any extraneous words. Put emotion-evoking words in it. Repeat it in your mind five times, and picture it in your mind each time you say it. Attempt to memorize it.
3. When you experience a trigger or feel a temptation to view or do, note it and keep track of the number of instances.

Whiteboard Chapter 6

"Where there is no vision, the people perish" (Prov. 29:18).

For your mind to see it clearly, your vision needs to be well-defined, vivid, and positive.

Add power to your vision by including emotion-evoking language and concrete, short-term benefits.

Vision Criteria:
- Does it paint a picture in your mind?
- Are the benefits of your vision directly yours, not others?
- Is it brief?
- Is it easy to say?
- Is it simple?

Note: *Please see samples and real-life visions of others and share your current vision at* poweroverpornography.com/vision

CHAPTER 7:

The Power of Acknowledging and Accepting

"Between stimulus and response there is a space. In that space is our power to choose our response. In our response lies our growth and our freedom."

Victor Frankl, *Man's Search for Meaning*

"Bailey, come here quickly," Jason shouted excitedly as soon as he stepped in the front door. He heard the familiar pitter-patter of her feet, one of his favorite sounds, as Bailey came running.

"Look what I found outside." Jason held up a big caterpillar. He knew Bailey loved bugs of all kinds and especially caterpillars. She jumped up and down and asked if she could hold it. "Of course," he replied.

Bailey grabbed the caterpillar eagerly but tenderly. She dashed into the kitchen, yelling, "Mom, can I have a jar? Look at the caterpillar Daddy bwung me. I need to put it in a jar with holes in the top so he can bwcathe."

Jason followed her into the kitchen. She was still jumping up and down, and the whole family started to feel her contagious excitement. "Hey, Mikey, how was school today? How about showing me your soccer skills after dinner?"

"Are you sure, Dad? You're usually too tired to play."

"I'm sure. I hear you can really kick the ball."

"I scored two goals at recess today."

"Great. Let's see what you've got!"

Jason glanced at Becky, who was just barely smiling. She was expressing some surprise as well. "Dinner won't be ready for fifteen minutes in case you two want to go outside now."

Mike's face lit up, and before she could finish her sentence, he dashed off to get his soccer ball. "Let's go, Dad," he yelled from the doorway.

Jason picked the baby, Nicole, up from her walker and gave her a big kiss. She smiled at him.

"So, Jason, how was your day today?" David asked as Jason arrived at the door for their next session.

"Great. I made a difference the other night with my kids after our session on vision, and I still feel good from it. I made it a goal to make each one feel happy, and I had some success. I decided to quit feeling sorry for myself and instead look for ways to help my children."

"Glad to hear it. We're going talk a little about feeling sorry for oneself as we cover the power of acknowledging and accepting today. Come in."

David kept talking as they entered the house and then the office. "I noticed you didn't say anything about how it went with your wife. Anything I should read into that?"

"I'm feeling a bit more love for her just from focusing on the consequences and my vision. I can see that the strained state of our marriage is my fault, not hers, but I don't know how to fix it. I still feel pretty bad about how my viewing has hurt our relationship and hurt her for so many years."

"I'm glad you're feeling more love for your wife and kids. I think as you continue in the program and work on getting your power back, you'll know how to begin realizing your vision with her.

"By the way, I didn't see you at the twelve-step meeting last night. Are you going to a different meeting?"

Jason looked a bit surprised. "I thought that I wouldn't need to go to those meetings now that I'm doing this program with you. Do I need to go?"

David responded with caring. "It's always your choice whether to go or not. I attend because of the healing power I feel from the group members who share, the strength I receive, and the strong spirit that is there. There is power in sharing and admitting our weaknesses, and although I've been sober from viewing for twenty-two years, I know that I'm still vulnerable."

Jason felt the same healing power, strength, and strong spirit just being with David, but as David spoke about the meetings, Jason felt the need to begin attending again. "I think I'll see you at the next one."

"Jason, I'm excited about today, and I'm excited about the happy mood you bring with you. We're going to talk about a simple but strong power that you may not have heard discussed this way before."

As Jason turned toward the front of the office, he noticed a quote written on the board.

Problems do not go away. They must be worked through or else they remain, forever a barrier to the growth and development of the spirit... The truth is that our finest moments are most likely to occur when we are feeling deeply uncomfortable, unhappy, or unfulfilled. For it is only in such moments, propelled by our discomfort, that we are likely to step out of our ruts and start searching for different ways or truer answers.
—M. Scott Peck

He thought David would explain the quote later, but he recognized the truth in it and felt some satisfaction in knowing that he was working through his problem instead of wishing it away.

David began without referencing the quote on the board. "One of our goals is to turn your unconscious choice to view into a conscious one. We need to switch your handling of the viewing and doing temptation from your reptilian brain to your logical brain; in the latter, there is a space between stimulus and response to weigh consequences. We began that process with one of the homework assignments from last session. Do you recall the assignment to note each time you experienced a temptation to view?"

"I did that assignment out of my commitment, but I didn't think it would be helpful." Jason spoke plainly with David. He was not used to sharing his thoughts so directly, but David made him feel comfortable sharing, even if what he said could be controversial.

"I didn't understand why I should note each time I was tempted. In fact, it seems like doing so just makes me dwell on it more, and that makes it more likely that I'll relapse. I'm not sure that it is helpful."

David smiled. He seemed to welcome Jason's thoughts even if they were contradictory. "Thanks for letting me know. Many people view it the same way. Today, you'll learn why noting the temptation is part of the program. You'll also get some additional tools that will provide you with tremendous power. Just bear with me as we cover some other important concepts first."

Jason nodded his acceptance.

"I'm going to start by asking you a question: how do you feel when you are tempted to view pornography?"

Jason didn't need to think long before he answered. These feelings had been on his mind since he started meeting with David. "I feel guilty and powerless. Once I feel the urge, it seems that viewing is inevitable because I'm weak. I also feel self-hatred start to creep into my thoughts because I'm weak. However, I started to feel more confident after the first lesson with you. Clarifying the consequences and establishing a vision have given me even more confidence that I can do this."

"I'm happy to hear that you're getting some of your confidence back. That is normal at this point in the program, but we still have some important concepts to learn and to apply. In fact, we need to put it all together so you have the complete toolset in a step-by-step formula. That will come soon, but for now, let's keep dealing with the temptation to view.

"Do you think that all people experience the same urges and temptations?" David asked.

"Probably, but some of the men at church seem like they have it together pretty well."

"You're right. Some do have it more together, but all men have problems and experience temptation. In fact, almost all men and most women experience the temptation to view or do. We often judge ourselves more harshly than we judge others; however, viewers are pretty harsh judges of others who have the same anger and lack-of-love issues.

"The best men in the world feel the urges and temptations that you feel, even those who seem to have it together. We want to work on disconnecting the urge with the pornography viewing itself. One way to do this is to recognize that all men have the same urges, even though we don't know the degree to which we each feel them."

David wrote on the whiteboard, "Temptations or urges are not bad" and "Temptations come to everyone."

"There is no reason to feel guilty or powerless when the temptation comes; as I've said, it comes to everyone, and it is just a thought with no power except the power we give it. The next time you experience temptation, tell yourself, 'This is just a thought (or feeling or temptation). It does not reflect on me because temptations come to everyone without exception. I need not feel guilty, shameful, powerless, or weak just because I feel tempted to view and do.'

"One of the ways we give our power away to temptation is by feeling guilt and shame when we experience it. Therefore, the first step in taking your power back is to realize that the temptation is not the source of the guilt and shame. The action we take after experiencing the temptation is the source."

"Hold on, David. I sometimes experience temptations to do some pretty awful things, and I doubt if others experience them in the same way or to the same extent. It's hard not to feel guilty and shameful when I feel tempted in this way."

"Jason, what specifically makes you feel that your temptations are different than what others experience, and what is it about those temptations that makes you feel guilty and shameful?"

"I'm embarrassed to tell you, but when I see a beautiful woman either in person or on TV, movies, or wherever, I often feel tempted to have sex with her. It may not be a realistic desire, but it's still the temptation. It seems wrong to have thoughts of being unfaithful to my wife."

"I appreciate your candor. It's certainly difficult to know the frequency and degree of strength of others' temptations, but I don't know if the temptation you've described is that different from what others experience. I encourage you to think of your temptation as merely a thought with no power. Think of this particular temptation as one that is common. You'll find this attitude will help you as we move into our next steps.

"Can you think of each temptation as just a thought with no power to make you feel shame or guilt?"

"I think so. The thought of treating it as a powerless thought that is common to many people is appealing. Maybe my guilt and shame is due to my behavior of almost always acting on the temptation in the past. So, when I feel the temptation, I also feel the emotions of acting on it because that's been the norm for me."

"Good thought. Let's continue. The second way we give our power to the temptation is to resist it."

Jason was surprised by this statement and blurted out, "What do you mean we give power to it by resisting it? Are you saying I should just succumb to it and view and do? That doesn't make any sense at all." Jason's voice was raised, and David detected some anger creeping into it.

David calmly replied, "It seems like you're feeling pretty feisty today, Jason. That's OK. The concepts are new to you. Your reaction is not unusual when someone first hears that resisting temptation takes power from us and gives it to the temptation. We've been taught all of our lives that we should resist temptations. It seems counterintuitive to now say someone should stop resisting."

Now Jason agreed. "Yeah, really counterintuitive."

"Try to suspend your inner skeptic for a moment while I walk you through how not resisting is different than succumbing and how resisting works against your taking control. Let's first discuss the principle and then get into practical ways to demonstrate its effectiveness."

David's words calmed Jason's emotions.

David continued, "Paraphrasing Stephen Covey, when we try to kill a feeling, it struggles for life. When we let it live, it dies birthing. The founder of modern psychology, Carl Jung reportedly stated it another way: 'What we resist, persists.'"

"In the past, you would commonly view and do upon experiencing the temptation. So naturally your focus has been on trying to avoid triggers and certain situations to limit experiencing temptation. You thought this would prevent you from viewing and doing. Let me state this as plainly as I can: this doesn't work.

"When you attempt to avoid or resist the temptation, it tracks you down and fights back."

Jason interrupted him here. "I still don't get it. I'm trying not to be skeptical, but what is the alternative to resisting aside from succumbing to the temptation?"

David smiled. "I'm glad you asked. There is a third alternative that is much more powerful than either resisting or succumbing. Let me walk you through it.

"The first step is to acknowledge the urge as plainly as possible. When we feel the temptation to view pornography, we deprive it of power by acknowledging it with a simple statement like, 'I want to look at pornography' or 'I want to look at pornography and masturbate.' Or, using our vocabulary, you would say, 'I want to view and do.' Referring to the temptation you mentioned, your acknowledgment would be, 'I want to have sex with that woman.'

"Practice this in your mind by repeating your most common viewing or doing temptation. Instead of trying to force the temptation out of your mind, let it live.

"Acknowledging the temptation is crucial to your success in this program. In fact, if you skip this step, you're not likely to succeed. You've probably been trying to resist the temptation for a long time. As Dr. Phil would ask, 'How has that worked out for you?'"

Jason wasn't sure about David's sense of humor but couldn't help smiling. "Not so great."

"Just like the purple hippo, when we try to resist or suppress the temptation to view pornography, it stays in our mind until we act on it or acknowledge it. Most viewers aren't used to acknowledging it; they believe the temptation itself is an expression of their own inadequacies or evil nature. By realizing temptation is natural and comes to everyone, it becomes easier to acknowledge.

"In other words, acknowledging temptation is crucial to success because it places you in control." David turned to write on the board:

"We give power to ourselves when we _____ acknowledge the temptation plainly, directly, and specifically."

"You've sparked my curiosity with the missing word," Jason remarked.

"I think you're beginning to see the power of acknowledging, but there is an important element that I left out, and I thought you may have fun trying to guess it."

Jason looked at the board and thought out loud, "Hmm. How about 'boldly?'"

"I like that. Maybe we'll have to add 'boldly' to the statement as well. But the answer has to do with timing."

"I would guess that you would want to address the temptation immediately."

"Correct. You win my congratulations. You seemed pretty sure about the need to acknowledge the temptation immediately. Why do you think that is important?"

"The purple hippo came to mind. I thought that the more time I let pass from when the temptation arrived, the more smashing the hippo would do. In other words, the more I let the temptation hang around without acknowledging it, the more likely I am to act on it."

"Great way to put it, Jason. Let me cover a couple of other important points. Earlier, when I asked you to practice acknowledging in your mind by repeating your most common viewing temptation, what did you think?"

"My thought was, 'I'm being tempted to view and do.'"

"If you change your wording, you'll take back even more power. Practice acknowledging temptation in a way that gives you responsibility.

In other words, starting the sentence with 'I want to…' means you're taking responsibility for the urge or temptation. Starting the sentence with 'I'm tempted to…' takes you off the hook a little by assigning the temptation to forces outside of you. Although the temptation may originate from outside of you, can you see the subtle difference and recognize how taking personal responsibility gives you more power?"

"I think so," Jason responded.

"You'll see it even more clearly as we go on.

"Let me emphasize another point that I alluded to earlier. Remember how we discussed the idea that temptation, particularly the viewing and doing temptation, comes to virtually all men?"

"Sure."

"The main reason I brought that up was to allow you to more easily accept the temptation once you acknowledge it. Some people acknowledge the temptation but still experience guilt over having it. They don't accept it as normal.

"As you see, the second important component of this lesson is accepting the temptation. Once you acknowledge the temptation, you accept it as normal—just a thought, something that everyone experiences. You acknowledge and accept it as occurring to you in that moment. The acceptance removes the guilt and shame and allows you to deal with the temptation at a conscious level.

"In the past, you've dealt with the temptation at a subconscious level, automatically reverting to the shame cycle reaction that meant, 'If I experience the temptation, then I view and do.' When you acknowledge and accept the temptation you unlink it from the action and can then deal with it consciously. Does that make sense?"

David turned to the whiteboard while waiting for Jason's response.

Jason appreciated that David checked to make sure he understood. "It does make sense. My skeptical self does not want to believe that merely acknowledging and accepting the temptation will solve the problem. But I can see how it is more effective than just moving right from temptation to action."

"That's all I'm asking for now. You're right that acknowledging and accepting alone won't solve the problem but when combined with the powers and tools we'll cover in the upcoming session, it will. During our next session, you'll learn how to use one of the greatest powers of the entire course."

Homework for Power of Acknowledging and Accepting:
1. Write your vision and state it five times. Remember, practice helps rewire your brain.
2. Acknowledge every temptation by stating it in terms that indicate personal responsibility, such as, "I want to view and do" or "I want to have sex with that person."
3. Accept each temptation as normal. Remind yourself that everyone experiences temptation, and it should not be directly associated with guilt or shame.

Whiteboard Chapter 7

Temptations or urges are not bad.

Temptations come to everyone.

We give power to ourselves when we:
- Immediately acknowledge the temptation plainly, directly, and specifically.
- Accept the temptation as normal, not unusual.
- Accept experiencing the temptation without shame or guilt.

Chapter 8:

The Power to Choose

"Another way we give power to temptation is to tell ourselves that we must not give in to it. When someone tells us we must not do something, we typically rebel. We don't like being compelled to do something by others or by ourselves.

"When you tell yourself you must not give in, you attempt to compel yourself to act in a certain way, depriving yourself of the freedom to choose. When you take the power away from yourself through statements that make you feel compelled, you give the power to the temptation. But remember, you always have the power to choose."

David turned to the whiteboard and wrote, "You always have a choice; you aren't required to do anything."

Jason was intrigued by this. He felt the truth and power of the statement even though he hadn't previously thought about it that way. He thought that he lacked self-discipline because he was not able to follow through when he told himself he must quit. Maybe he was just rebelling against a statement of force. When he told himself that he must not give in, he was rarely able to get the temptation out of his mind and almost always succumbed to it.

As usual, it seemed like David read his mind. "When you say 'must' or 'have to,' you give your power to the temptation, and you're rarely able to overcome it. In fact, I like to refer to these words that try to force us to do something as the 'MuHa lie.'

"When you tell yourself you must or you have to do something, you're lying to yourself. You don't have to do anything. You always have a choice. Even a prisoner can choose not to follow orders. He or she might suffer severe consequences, but the choice is still there.

"Whenever you tell yourself that you must or must not do something or that you have to do something, just laugh with a deep muhaha! Combining the m-u from 'must' and the h-a from 'have to' is a fun and effective way to remember this. It will remind you that you just lied to yourself and tried to take away your right to choose."

Jason couldn't help but laugh when he heard David try his deep MuHa laugh. As Jason laughed and practiced a MuHa laugh, David wrote on the board, "Catch the MuHa lie."

"Whenever you hear yourself saying any of the following phrases in a sentence, stop and tell yourself it's a lie: I must, I must not, I have to, I can't, I've got to. Change your language to 'I choose to...'

"Another important concept of free choice is the ability to change choices. If, when you make a choice, you are required to stick with that choice for the rest of your life, then you've taken away all future choices. This is against the nature of free choice.

"If you make choices that can't be changed in the future, what have you done to your power to choose?"

Jason was confused. "I thought that commitment was an important part of overcoming pornography, so I guess you have to make the choice to live a loving life, and then your future choices will be limited."

"What does that do to your future freedom to choose?"

"It takes it away."

"The next time the temptation to view and do hits you, what do you tell yourself if that's your perspective?"

"I guess you would tell yourself that you can't view because you exercised your choice some time ago."

"I think you're right. If you made the choice once, then you would resort to MuHa in the future. However, this goes against the nature of your freedom, and it causes you to rebel against yourself. The likely result would be that you would feel deprived because you no longer had a choice.

"Once you start feeling deprived, you feel like a victim, and you use victim language and feel sorry for yourself. Then you're left with fighting the temptation instead of accepting it and choosing your actions. This cycle almost always ends in succumbing to temptation.

"So, as much as we would like to make the choice once and limit all future choices, it doesn't work. After you feel like a victim, you may think you deserve to view, and if you act on this, you're right back into the miserable cycle of viewing and doing, feeling guilty, resolving not to do it again, feeling deprived, feeling the need to view, and so on."

Jason thought that this made sense, but he wasn't sure how to maintain a commitment and his freedom to choose at the same time. "What is the solution?"

"The solution is the simple truth that every decision you make is momentary. You make a decision for this instance and no other. You reserve the right to choose differently in all future instances.

"This solution does not deny your prior commitment, but it tells the basic truth that you can always choose to violate that commitment, and so you maintain the freedom to choose your actions no matter what the circumstances are."

"It seems like having to make the decision every time you're faced with temptation would work against you."

David smiled. "I know it may seem like that, but as we put it all together, you'll see how it is the only way to preserve your freedom to choose. This is one of the greatest powers you have and of this entire program. One of my favorite quotations that illustrates the importance of this God-given power is, 'Next to the bestowal of life itself, the right to direct that life is God's greatest gift to man....Freedom of choice is more to be treasured than any possession earth can give.'[ii]

"When you give yourself the freedom to choose differently in the future, how can you feel deprived? You're only choosing for this instance, so you're free to view and do upon the next temptation if you wish to.

"The power you get from this freedom is often the same power that you long ago gave to the temptation, often with the thought, 'This is the last time.' But it never was. Your freedom to choose differently was gone. The time has come to take it back, and you're almost there.

"I believe that choosing once in the form of a commitment can help us establish what we want in life, and we can then make choices that are consistent with getting there. However, we succeed when we are free to choose each time.

"I also tend to believe that those who are not addicted can choose once and then just reconfirm that decision upon future temptations. But it doesn't work like that for addicts. Maybe it's because we've tried and failed so many times at long-term commitments, and we know subconsciously that doing so again is a failure path. Regardless of the reason, realizing that we are free to choose differently every time gives us power.

"In summary," David stated as he wrote on the whiteboard, "Every choice is for this instance only. When we try to make our choices permanent, we take away our right to decide in the future. This feels like compelling ourselves to make a certain decision."

He continued, "Let's get back to the idea of compulsion and using language of force. We just learned that we naturally rebel against compulsion even when it comes from ourselves. Let's review and expand that a little more before discussing other elements of the power of free choice.

"What are some of the phrases we use to try to compel ourselves to take certain actions, stop thinking specific thoughts, or to change our behavior?"

Jason recalled the MuHa acronym and how it was present in his self-talk. "'I must do it' or 'I must not think these thoughts' are probably my most common statements. I also tell myself 'I have to do this.'"

"I think these are very common. Can you think of any other ways we try to compel ourselves to action? Think of some of the ways your parents may have tried to talk you into doing or not doing something when you were a teenager."

"When my dad was mad, he would usually say, 'You'd better not.' My mother would usually say things like, 'You should clean your room' or 'You should do this or should not do that.'"

"Good. You've listed four ways we use language to compel ourselves to do something: MuHa and now BS for 'better' and 'should.' I don't care for the acronym BS, so I added another letter in the middle: O stands for 'ought to.' Often we tell ourselves that we ought to or ought not to do something.

"Another common way we try to compel ourselves to do something is when we say 'supposed to,' such as, 'I'm not supposed to eat cookies before dinner' or "I'm not supposed to browse or look at the files on another person's computer' or 'I know I'm supposed to go to bed now, but this TV show is too good to turn off.' The phrase 'supposed to' produces the same feelings as the words 'better' and 'should.' We feel compelled, and we naturally rebel. Now the acronym is BOSS, which fits quite nicely. When we use 'better,' 'ought to,' 'should,' or 'supposed to,' we're making them the boss instead of leaving the bossing to ourselves and using our own power to choose.

"In addition to the MuHa laugh, now you have the BOSS acronym to catch yourself when you say things like you'd better not or should not view, or when you say you ought to or you're supposed to or you ought not or you're not supposed to. Whenever we use these or similar phrases, we are trying to compel ourselves to do something, and our mind will not cooperate." You have the choice, so when you tell yourself these things, immediately follow it up with a rousing 'They're not the boss!'

Jason liked the acronyms. They were funny and useful. While Jason chuckled to himself, David wrote, "BOSS (better, ought to, should, or supposed to) is not the boss," on the whiteboard.

David kept writing as he spoke, "As we mentioned previously, one of the ways we gain power is to make our unconscious habits into conscious choices. This is directly connected to the use of language that tries to compel. Instead of saying, 'I must go to bed right now,' we can say, 'I choose to go to bed right now.' An important part of the program and getting your power back is to always recognize and exercise your power to choose.

"Sometimes this is a tough recognition for viewers to make. They grasp the concept but have a harder time translating it into action."

"What do you mean?"

"Let me illustrate. During the growing months, I typically mow my lawn every Saturday afternoon. I can tell myself, 'It's Saturday afternoon, so I must mow the grass.' This is a force statement that takes away my power to choose. I don't really have to mow my lawn. I can choose not to. What are the consequences of choosing not to mow?"

"Your grass gets long, your neighbors complain, you're embarrassed of your yard, and it becomes harder to mow the next time."

"Those are logical consequences of not mowing, but the choice is mine. No one is forcing me to mow.

"Often, those who have a strong sense of duty to their tasks—and that strong sense of duty is a good thing—can have a difficult time putting the concept of choice into practice. What do you think?"

"As an accountant, I tend to have a strong sense of duty, and I haven't really thought of my actions as choices. It may take effort for me to implement this, but it feels right, so I'm excited to try."

"Great. Let's move a little deeper."

Jason was a little surprised that David moved on despite his wishy-washy answer. But he now trusted David completely and relaxed his inner skeptic almost immediately.

David continued, "We discussed earlier how important it is to acknowledge and accept the temptation when it comes to you and to be specific. In the next breath after doing so, exercise your freedom to choose. The more deliberate, plain, and direct your expression of your freedom to choose, the more power you retain to make the choice.

David went back to the board. "I know some of this is repetitive, but I think it's important to solidify the concept and its application, so I'll write it a bit differently this time."

"For example, when you're tempted to view pornography, state to yourself, 'I want to look at pornography.' You accept that temptation as normal and then recognize your choice by saying to yourself, 'And I'm free to choose.' By recognizing and exercising the choice, you've taken the power back from the temptation."

"Let's discuss another element of the power of choosing. We discussed this extensively in an earlier session, but it fits in here as well. When we choose benefits or consequences, we give ourselves power. By deliberately stating our choice as one of benefits, consequences, and vision, the power of that choice becomes real.

"For example, if I don't like to run, bike, or exercise in some other way, but I have a vivid vision of having high energy and enjoying the benefits of being in shape, then my choice to run becomes easier. In essence, I don't say to myself 'I want to run.' This is a deceptive way of trying to compel myself to run.

"Instead, I say to myself, 'I choose to have the energy to play with my kids for a few hours, and I choose to look great and feel proud of my body.' This vision is truthful, and it focuses on the positive results. Choosing a vision full of positive consequences is more powerful than the temptation."

David added another bullet to the board that said, "Choosing a vision with positive results gives you power."

"Does this make sense to you, Jason?"

"It's starting to make a lot of sense. I like the way the choice is not about viewing or not viewing but about choosing the positive consequences."

"Great. We'll be getting into choosing your vision a little more next session. The next session is when it all comes together. You'll come away with a concrete plan of action for dealing with temptation. I can tell you're feeling the power of the concepts, but you'll feel the real power of the program when it all comes together.

"Don't forget your homework. I'll see you next time."

Homework for the Power to Choose:

1. Write the following statements. After each statement, practice the MuHa laugh.
   a. I must not view.
   b. I must not do.
   c. I have to be good.
   d. I must go to bed on time.
   e. I have to mow the lawn.
2. Write the following statements. After each statement, practice saying, "You're not the boss of me."
   a. I'd better not view.
   b. I should not do.
   c. I'd better stay off my computer tonight.
   d. I should clean the bathroom.
   e. I'm supposed to go out tonight.
   f. I ought to turn off the computer.
3. Practice saying, "I choose to..." whenever you would normally use compelling or force language. When you catch yourself using "must," "have to" (MuHa), "better," "ought," "should," "supposed to" (BOSS), or any other language of force, such as "can't," or "got to," tell yourself it is a lie. You are not required to do anything. It is your choice. You always have the freedom to choose.
4. Write and then say, "I always have a choice, and my choice is for this instance only. I can choose differently in the next instance." Practice this three more times before the next session.
5. Write and then say, "When I choose, I choose a vision and its consequences, not just action." Repeat this three times before the next session.

Whiteboard Chapter 8-1

You always have a choice; you aren't required to do anything.

Catch the MuHa lie.

Every choice is for this instance only.

BOSS (better, ought to, should, supposed to) is not the boss.

Make unconscious habits into conscious choices.

Whiteboard Chapter 8-2

Power in Free Choice
- Choices are momentary, not permanent. You are free to choose differently next time.
- Compelling ourselves results in rebellion. You naturally rebel against MuHa and BOSS.
- Deliberately acknowledging your right to choose gives you power.
- Choosing a vision with positive results gives you power.

CHAPTER 9:

The Power of Acknowledge and Accept, Choose, and Vision (AACV) Together

When Jason parked in his driveway that night, he felt tired. Work had been taxing, and he felt emotionally drained after the session at David's house. He wanted to sit in front of the TV for an hour just to recover. Jason caught himself, realizing that he was not just choosing actions; he was choosing consequences. He was letting his lazy mind dictate his actions, disregarding the consequences. Maybe the consequences were a little cloudy.

He turned toward the power to choose quickly. He thought, *Regardless of how I feel or how I'm tempted to act, I can choose how I respond. Choosing a loving life will help me realize my vision, and choosing my reactions to other temptations, like sitting in front of the TV instead of helping Becky or playing with the kids, will also help me realize my vision.*

His plan to greet his kids with a weary look faded completely as he chose to act lively and to help or play. By exercising his freedom to choose, the feeling of tiredness left, just like the temptation to view and do left when he chose a vision of positive consequences.

Jason expected to be greeted with smiling, happy kids and a smiling, happy wife when he walked in the door. Instead, he found emptiness except for some loud banging noises coming from the kitchen. He strode quickly toward these sounds.

Becky was furiously fixing dinner, banging pots on the counter with gusto. Jason felt an urge to tiptoe away but stayed and asked, "What's wrong, Becky?"

As soon as Becky turned to him, Jason regretted asking. "Your children are in their rooms," Becky said quickly and loudly. "Michael broke a lamp, Bailey is nursing a bloody nose and falling asleep, and Nicole exhausted herself from the commotion and is sleeping as well."

Jason could tell that their sleeping had taken a great deal of effort on Becky's part. She continued, "Your son decided to play soccer in the family room and asked Bailey to be the goalie. He kicked the ball so hard that it bounced off her nose and hit the lamp."

Jason felt a little pride in hearing how hard Mike kicked the ball, but he quickly hid that thought and moved closer to Becky. He could tell she was ready to cry, but she continued. "I finally stopped the blood from Bailey's nose. Nicole was screaming because Bailey was screaming. Once Bailey calmed down and wanted to go lay in her bed, I held Nicole until she fell asleep. I didn't even get a chance to yell at Mike because he went straight to his room. I told him you would talk to him tonight."

This is the point that Jason would normally have started talking about how rough his day was, trying to one-up Becky. He felt the temptation but caught himself and responded to her story. "I'm sorry it was so hectic for you. I'll talk to Mike in a little while. Are you OK?"

Jason moved to hug Becky and she almost lunged into his arms, holding him tightly and crying. "I'm fine, just a little wound up. I didn't really like that lamp anyway." The tears turned to laughter, and they both smiled. She let go and said, "Let me finish getting dinner ready while you go talk to Mr. Indoor Soccer."

Jason kissed her and went to talk with Mike. As he was going upstairs, he thought about how he was changing a little. He felt love for his wife that he had not felt for her in months. He was concerned for her, and this warmed his heart. He had listened to her and felt like he responded halfway decently. Maybe he could make this work after all.

Jason had a short conversation with Mike, who was faking sleep when Jason first entered his room. Rather than getting angry, Jason complimented Mike on his leg strength, repeated the rule about no soccer in the house, and helped Mike plan his apologies to his mom and Bailey. He arranged a payment plan for Mike to pay off the lamp. Jason set the lamp value at a discounted ten dollars. Becky's comment about not liking the lamp probably saved Mike twenty dollars. Jason also offered to play goalie for Mike outside after dinner.

"Welcome back, Jason. Today is the most important day of the program. We are going to put together the four vital elements." As David spoke, he wrote these statements on the board, "Acknowledge the temptation, accept the temptation as normal, exercise your power to choose, and choose your vision of positive consequences."

"These four elements are the foundation of the program and sources of your power to live a loving life. Let me illustrate.

"We can return to my running choice as an example. I would tell myself, 'I don't want to run (acknowledge the urge or temptation), and that's OK (accept the temptation as normal), but I'm free to choose (exercise your power to choose), and I choose to have the energy to play with my kids for hours and to look great (choose the vision of positive consequences).'

"When you say this to yourself, do you feel compelled or deprived of your couch potato status?"

"No, but I enjoy running, so it's hard for me to feel that way for this example. Even so, I see your point, and I believe that I would not feel compelled or deprived if I didn't like to run."

"Jason, why don't you make it more real by making a similar statement regarding your viewing temptation?"

"OK, I'll give it a try: I want to view pornography...and I'm free to choose, and I choose to, um, let me see..." Jason turned to his notebook and read his vision. "I choose to show my deep love for my wife and kids by hugging, laughing, listening, talking, and spending time together doing what we like and confidently initiating and completing work that exceeds expectations."

"Do you feel compelled not to view pornography? Do you feel denied or deprived that you can't look at pornography?"

"No. It feels very empowering and freeing. I know that I can choose to view pornography whenever I want, but it feels good to choose the vision. I smile when I think of my family smiling, and I no longer feel the urge running around in my mind or the guilt and shame that come with it."

"Great. Like we discussed before, when you openly and honestly acknowledge the temptation, it loses power. When you try to kill it, suppress it, avoid it, substitute something else for it, or let it linger, it gains power.

"Let's make it a little more real by putting it in writing." David turned to modify the writing on the whiteboard until it said, "I want to view pornography. I accept this temptation as real and normal, and I am free to choose. I choose to show my deep love for my wife and kids by hugging, laughing, listening, talking, and spending time together doing what we like and confidently initiating and completing work that exceeds expectations."

"We should also discuss the power of the written word. Any idea what I mean by that?"

"Do you mean inspirational books that help motivate us and keep us on the right track?"

"No, but I think that is an excellent idea. When I read scripture or other inspirational books, my motivation and my personal power increase. I've often thought that this type of reading strengthens the power of my vision."

Jason thought that he would read his scriptures more regularly and try reading other inspirational books, but he was still curious about what David was referring to. "I agree, but you said no. What did you mean by the power of the written word?"

"Thanks for getting me back on track, Jason. Let me focus by reciting one of my favorite sayings, 'A goal not written is merely a wish.' Have you heard that before?"

"I have. You mentioned it in our first meeting, and I think it's a part of every goal-setting program my company has ever introduced."

"This idea is fundamental to the success of this program, which is really goal-setting as well. In fact, success in this program is essential to setting and achieving goals in other parts of your life. Without overcoming viewing and doing, your ability to achieve in any other area of your life is reduced substantially.

"We use the power of the written word to help you remember the four-step AACV, and I recommend you write it and refer to it often. By the way, POP stands for 'Power over Pornography,' and AACV stands for 'acknowledge, accept, choose, and vision': acknowledge (the temptation), accept (the temptation), exercise your freedom to choose, and choose the vision.

"I hope you don't mind all my acronyms. I find they make it easier to remember the key concepts, and the AACV is the critical part of the program. I'm sorry it's not as catchy as MuHa, BOSS, or POP, but hopefully it will help you remember the key steps in dealing with temptation directly."

David grabbed a note card from the shelf and handed it to Jason. "While we have your specific four-step AACV on the board, why don't you write it on the card so you can take it with you?

"You may be worried about someone else finding the card, so you may wish to write in code. Many people with a viewing and doing addiction can become so concerned about others finding out that they don't follow the program. Following the program is vital to your recovery, so we want to take away that fear." David wrote on the board: "I want to V (and D), a real and normal temptation. I am free to choose, and I choose deep love for my wife and kids by hugging, laughing, listening, talking, and spending time and being praised for my work, exceeding expectations."

"I changed the wording of the vision slightly to make it shorter, but it still captures the meaning. I recommend shortening it as much as you can so it becomes hard to forget. But it's your vision, so feel free to change it back."

Jason didn't respond, so David kept talking. "You now have the fundamental building blocks to deal with temptation directly and to choose a higher vision. My guess is that you're feeling the power of these building blocks, and you may even feel confident.

"Confidence is essential to living a loving life and a productive, happy life. But there is a downside to it that I want to cover.

"Some people feel confident enough at this stage that they believe they are ready to leave the program. I always urge them not to because there are still some vital concepts to learn and practice before they're ready to move on. The word 'practice' will take on additional meaning and power in a future session. The next session will show you four powerful ways that you've given your power away and what you can do to get it back.

"It's getting late. Let's end for today with your homework. I'm interested in talking to you next time about how this works for you."

Homework for the Power of AACV:

1. When you catch yourself using "must," "have to" (MuHa), "better," "ought to," "should," "supposed to" (BOSS), or any other language of force, such as "can't," or "got to," tell yourself it is a lie. You don't have to, and you are not required to. It is your choice. You always have the freedom to choose.
2. Practice the four-part approach to dealing with the temptation to view and do:
   a. Acknowledge the urge or temptation.
   b. Accept it as real and normal.
   c. Recognize and exercise your right and power to choose.
   d. Choose the vision and positive consequences of living a loving life.

3. Write your personalized four-step POP AACV "Acknowledge, Accept, Choose, Vision," phrases in specific language on a three-by-five note card and read it every time you're tempted. This is a very important part of the program.

Whiteboard Chapter 9-1

- Acknowledge the temptation.
- Accept the temptation as normal.
- Exercise your power to choose.
- Choose your vision of positive consequences.

Whiteboard Chapter 9-2

- I want to view pornography.
- I accept this temptation as real and normal.
- I am free to choose.
- I choose to show my deep love for my wife and kids by hugging, laughing, listening, talking, and spending time together doing what we like and confidently initiating and completing work that exceeds expectations.

Note: *You can find a pre-formatted AACV card to print and carry with you at* poweroverpornography.com/AACVcard.

CHAPTER 10:

The Power of Stress, Anxiety, and Discomfort

Jason climbed slowly out of the car, still trying to put together the pieces of the evening with David. This was the day he had been waiting for—the step-by-step formula to overcome his viewing. He thought he would feel great on this day, but instead, he felt anxiety about his failed past and its meaning to his future.

Would this program really help him overcome his addiction? So far, he agreed with everything David had taught him, but he was nervous now that he was actually committed to implementing the program.

Maybe the thought of leaving behind the viewing is making me nervous Jason thought as he entered the house. He tried to put on his game face to play with the kids and treat Becky right. Becky looked tired and irritated, and the kids seemed to have swallowed some wild pills.

After struggling through the evening, battling his own anxiety, and trying to figure out why he wasn't connecting with Becky or the kids, Jason checked his e-mail. He felt the temptation to view coming to him when he opened up the browser, but he was prepared. He read his AACV card and then signed into his e-mail account.

He focused on stating the temptation out loud in his mind and accepting it—it was OK to experience this temptation. He then said in his mind, *I am free to choose*, followed by, *and I choose to show my deep love for my wife and kids by hugging, laughing, listening, talking, and spending time doing what we like and confidently initiating and completing work that exceeds expectations.*

Hey, maybe this is going to work after all, he thought as the temptation left him. The seriousness of the consequences along with the thoughts to acknowledge and accept had kept him free from viewing since he started the program. Now he was feeling a little more confident that he could do this.

As soon as Jason sat down in David's office for their next session, David looked at him, smiled, and asked, "How did it go?"

"It went great. The formula works."

"I'm glad to hear that you had a good experience implementing the steps of the program. Did you feel any stress or anxiety?"

"You must be a mind reader. I had some anxious moments that I didn't expect. I enjoyed each session and felt the truth and effectiveness of what you said, so the pit in my stomach took me by surprise."

"I'm not much of a mind reader, but anxiety, stress, and discomfort are part of the program. Don't get worried. Kahlil Gibran, a poet and visual artist said, 'Comfort, that stealthy thing that enters the house a guest, and then becomes a host, then a master. And then it becomes a tamer, and with a hook and whip it makes puppets of your larger desires.'

"I like this quote because it lets us know that if we're feeling too comfortable, we may not be accomplishing our larger desires. Have you ever discussed the notion of a comfort zone before?"

"Sure, we talk about it all the time at work. For example, we talk about getting out of our comfort zones to talk to hard clients, deliver bad news, and things like that."

David smiled and said, "We have to get out of our comfort zones to achieve any worthy objective, especially if it involves overcoming a problem. The longer the problem has been with us, the greater the comfort zone we've developed around it, and the more anxious we feel when we think about leaving that comfort zone.

"I think the following quote by Scott Peck illustrates it well." David pointed to the board and read the quote posted there.

Problems do not go away. They must be worked through or else they remain, forever a barrier to the growth and development of the spirit… The truth is that our finest moments are most likely to occur when we are feeling deeply uncomfortable, unhappy, or unfulfilled. For it is only in such moments, propelled by our discomfort, that we are likely to step out of our ruts and start searching for different ways or truer answers.
—*M. Scott Peck*

"It doesn't address the comfort zone as plainly as I like to discuss it, but it makes the point that discomfort is part of choosing a better way. Overcoming a long-held habit like viewing, although easier in this program than in most, still involves some discomfort."

Jason looked disappointed. "I guess I didn't realize that there would be some anxiety, given the steps you described."

"Let me tell you how powerful stress, anxiety, and discomfort can be for you."

"Do you mean how powerful it can be in causing me to view and do?"

"No, but I'm glad you brought it up. In the past, what was your reaction to stress, anxiety, or discomfort?"

"I would often view and do when I had these feelings. In fact, often is probably too mild a description. I can't think of many instances that viewing was not my answer to try to relieve stress."

"Did it solve your stress?"

"I always thought it did, but now that I think about it, the answer is no. I felt relief for a very short while, but the guilt, shame, and other negative consequences we discussed before just added to the stress, actually making it worse than it was before."

"This is the power of stress, anxiety, and discomfort. If you embrace them, welcome them, and accept them as the temporary result of your new life of love, they can be a powerful ally. After a few short weeks of experiencing them, your comfort zone expands, and the life of love starts to become yours.

"Let's talk about the comfort zone and the damage it can do in keeping you in the cycle of viewing and doing.

"You mentioned a key point I would like to discuss in a little more depth. You said that viewing and doing actually made the stress worse than it was before. Here's how that cycle works: You feel stress, anxiety, or discomfort, or maybe all three.

"In fact, let's use another acronym for this: SAD. It has a different meaning than the word 'sad,' so let's make sure we keep that in mind.

"In the past, when you felt SAD, you tried to get rid of the SAD by viewing and doing. The result of the viewing and doing was guilt, shame, and other negative consequences, and this made you feel more SAD. When you felt more SAD, you tried to get rid of it by viewing and doing, and on and on the cycle goes.

"Can you see how the way you dealt with your feelings of SAD in the past put you and kept you in the viewing and doing cycle?"

Jason sensed the truth of this and recalled how he justified his past viewing by thinking, *I'm feeling so stressed out. Viewing is a better alternative than going out looking for sex or than getting mad at someone.* That attitude only led to more stress so he was in the cycle. "Yeah. I can see how dealing with stress by viewing only keeps one in the viewing-doing and SAD cycle."

"Good. Let's dive a little deeper. In the past, you felt SAD, and then automatically, without thinking about consequences, you jumped into the cycle.

"What if, instead of seeking relief for the SAD, you decided to experience it fully? Let's look again at part of Scott Peck's quote. It says, 'Our finest moments are most likely to occur when we are feeling deeply uncomfortable, unhappy, or unfulfilled. For it is only in such moments, propelled by our discomfort, that we are likely to step out of our ruts and start searching for different ways or truer answers.'

"If we realize that feeling 'uncomfortable, unhappy, or unfulfilled,' or SAD, is a precursor to stepping out of our rut, then we can embrace the SAD instead of looking for ways to relieve it.

"This is the essence of the power of stress, anxiety, and discomfort: when we embrace these feelings, we grow outside of our comfort zone.

"Therefore, all we have to do is embrace the feelings of SAD as we realize that we are changing for the better and that it's OK to feel SAD and not do anything about it. Realize that the feelings are temporary; they last just a few days or weeks until our comfort zone grows big enough to encompass them.

"So, when you feel SAD now, take heart that you're stepping out of your rut and beginning the path toward living a loving life."

Jason reflected on this aloud. "I've never viewed stress quite this way before, but it seems logical. It's a little like acknowledging and accepting the temptation, but this time I'm acknowledging and accepting the feelings of SAD."

David agreed and started assigning Jason his homework.

Homework for the Power of Discomfort:

1. Embrace the feelings of stress, anxiety and discomfort. Realize that they are helping you expand your comfort zone and step out of your rut. Also realize that they will diminish over the next few days and weeks. Repeat the following when you feel SAD: "I feel stress. I am OK with feeling it because I know that I'm expanding my comfort zone and stepping out of my rut on the way to living a loving life."
2. Continue to use the AACV card for any temptations. Don't fall into the trap of letting the temptation linger; address it immediately by pulling the card out and reading it.

CHAPTER 11:

Giving away Your Power with SAPS

David started off their next meeting by saying, "During our last session, we talked about the power of stress, anxiety, and discomfort (SAD) and how the negative connotations of these feelings can be misplaced. When we embrace them as part of our growth toward expanding our comfort zone, then they can be powerful allies.

"You often experienced other emotions that led you to view and do in the past. Today, we're going to talk about how tying these feelings and emotions to viewing and doing is a lie that takes away your power. We're then going to discuss how to get that power back.

"First, we'll discuss the four main ways we give our power to viewing and how we can take that power back. Some of what we cover may sound familiar. We've alluded to a few of the concepts but haven't pointed them out as clearly as we will today.

"Before we move on to the four power takers, let's do an exercise. It may get a little personal, but I think you'll find it worthwhile.

"Please think about the last several times you succumbed to the temptation to view pornography. What were the feelings you had just prior to being tempted and giving in to it?"

Jason thought briefly. "Stress, anger at Becky, and ravenous but not for food—you know what I mean. I also felt bored, depressed, deprived of sex, or just nothing at all. I'm sure there are a lot of other feelings, but those are the ones that come to mind."

"Do you agree with the following statement: the reason you reached for pornography when you felt this way is because you initially chose to act and react that way."

"I think so. In the past, I felt like the choice was taken away from me. I would resolve to stop, but then I would still view the next time. That makes it feel less like a choice. But I'm pretty sure that the first time I chose to view and do as a response to any of those feelings, it was my choice."

"Once you made that first choice and then chose subsequently—whether consciously or not—to repeat the actions of viewing and doing, it became a natural response. I'm glad you realize that you're responsible and if you blame the stress, anger, boredom, depression, and so on for your choice to view pornography, you give your power away.

"One of the greatest ways to retain power is to take complete responsibility for our choices. Conversely, one of the greatest ways to lose power is to blame something or someone else.

"Whenever you start thinking about the reasons you gave in the past for viewing pornography, recognize that they are not valid reasons. You've trained yourself to view pornography when you experience those feelings."

David wrote, "Take responsibility for our choices and actions," on the whiteboard.

"Now, let's move on to the big four. We discussed in a prior session how resisting the temptation does not work. This is a key principle in understanding the four power takers. They have similar effects to resisting.

"In addition to trying to resist temptation in the past, you've likely tried to suppress it instead of acknowledging and accepting it. Suppression is the first of the big four power takers. It works similarly to resisting and has similar results, meaning it doesn't work."

Jason asked, "What is the difference between resisting and suppressing?"

David replied, "The difference in impact and result is very similar, but there is a difference. Some people really fight against the temptations, resisting them with a fighting spirit. Others do not want to fight but feel guilty and afraid of succumbing to the temptation, so they try to not think about it or try to suppress the thought. I hope that makes sense."

"Sure. I see the small difference and how they are very similar in result."

"What we try to suppress struggles for our attention until it receives it. It can receive it by our acknowledgment and acceptance or if we succumb to it.

"Suppressing the temptation does not work because we're abdicating responsibility for dealing with it, and we think that it will eventually go away if we try to ignore or suppress it. However, we know that if we don't deal with it, it will hang around until we succumb to it. We'll represent suppression with the first S in our SAPS acronym."

David wrote, "Tried and true failure paths: the power takers." Underneath it, he wrote, "Suppress the temptation."

"Let's move on to the second power taker. Some of the feelings you mentioned experiencing before you chose to view pornography would be identified by professional therapists as trigger emotions. Many of these professionals would recommend that you avoid the actions, circumstances, or places that lead to these emotions. Have you heard this before?"

"I've heard of triggers before, and I've tried to stay away from things that cause boredom and stress because I thought they tend to trigger my choices to view and do."

David smiled when he heard the word 'choices.'

Jason continued, "I've read that HALT is an acronym for some triggers. I believe it stands for hungry, angry, lonely, and tired. Whenever you feel these emotions or sensations, you should be on guard that you may slip. I think there is a lot of truth to that.

"I've been counseled before to not put myself in situations where I'll feel hungry, angry, lonely, or tired. The counselor told me to fill my time with worthwhile and wholesome activities so that the HALT feelings are kept at bay.

"Just recently, I heard a new acronym related to triggers. BLAST stands for bored, lonely, angry, stressed, and tired."

David seemed to ignore Jason's comments and stated, "Let me tell you something different about triggers. The very act of avoiding them and the temptations that follow takes power from you and gives it to your pornography viewing. Do you really think you'll always be able to avoid being hungry, angry, lonely, tired, bored, or stressed?"

Jason was a little shocked by this. It was the opposite of what he expected. "I haven't thought about that before, but I guess you're right. Now that I think about it, these feelings and situations are part of living, so they probably can't always be avoided. And if they can't, what do I do?"

"Before we discuss the answer, let's add another dimension to avoiding triggers. When we're addicted, new triggers and associated temptations will pop up unexpectedly. Or trigger circumstances will be bigger than us and thus unavoidable.

"Now, let's answer your question about what to do regarding triggers. Problems don't get solved by avoiding them. They get solved by confronting them. When you try to avoid triggers and their associated temptations or try to avoid the temptations directly, you aren't dealing with them, so they only get bigger the next time they arise. And they will arise again."

David turned to the whiteboard and added, "Avoid triggers and temptations."

"Don't get me wrong. I don't mean that you should deliberately subject yourself to triggers and temptations. But unless you learn to confront and deal with them, you'll eventually fail at living a loving life.

"In addition, avoiding triggers and their associated temptations is becoming less and less feasible. Scantily clad models are displayed on billboards or shown in commercials; these images are becoming increasingly brazen and acceptable. Nudity is becoming more acceptable on television programs as well, especially late-night television. And you know how easy it is to stumble upon nude images on the Internet.

"In many cases, avoiding these types of triggers is virtually impossible. You've now learned how to deal with them in a healthy, head-on way that works.

"Let's move on to the next popular way of trying to battle viewing and doing as well as many other addictions; this method is also destined to fail.

"One reason I switched to attending twelve-step meetings sponsored by the church I attend is that they don't allow smoking on their premises. I am not a smoker, and it has always bothered me that so much smoking goes on at some of the meetings. It seems that many alcoholics trade their alcohol addiction for a smoking addiction. I don't want to pass judgment on them because I think alcohol destroys lives more completely and quickly than smoking, but I think they give too much of their power away."

"What do you mean?"

"When we substitute one addiction for another, we're postponing our problem, just like avoidance. We're not dealing directly with the temptation. Substitution merely gives the temptation more power, taken directly from us."

"I understand an alcoholic substituting tobacco, but I'm not sure how and what I substitute for pornography."

"Let me give you an example. Some have suggested that using scripture verses or thinking of an uplifting hymn or song, even singing or humming it to oneself, can be a way of overcoming the temptation to view pornography. I believe that if this becomes part of your vision and you remember to exercise your choice, then it can be effective. If you are not addicted and are in prevention mode, it can also be effective.

"However, if you merely substitute reciting a song in your mind for the temptation, it hasn't really been dealt with and will come back, even if you experience temporary relief."

Jason was puzzled. "I think I'm beginning to understand. I've actually tried substituting a hymn for the temptation before, and it is usually a battle. I hum or sing the hymn in my mind, willing the temptation to go away. The temptation battles to come back, and if the hymn wins, it seems to be only a temporary win, like you said. The temptation is just under the surface and tends to come back pretty quickly. Then the battle starts all over again. Eventually the temptation wins."

"So, Jason, you've experienced the problem with substitution first-hand. You may win temporarily, but when the temptation hasn't been dealt with directly, it lingers and comes back often, sometimes more powerfully than before."

David turned to the whiteboard and added the additional failure path, "Substitute another thought or action."

"So, we see that substitution is a common practice that doesn't work. Can you think of other ways you may have tried to use substitution in the past?"

Jason thought for a moment before saying, "One of the programs I tried seemed to rely wholly upon substitution. The goal was to fill up my life with so many activities, primarily exercise and wholesome activities, that I wouldn't have time or attention available for the temptation.

"I think exercise is good for you, but it didn't keep me away from falling to the temptation. I also tried meditating, scripture reading, prayer, reading uplifting literature, and many other things. I can't argue with most of them; they're good for you, but I can confirm that substitution doesn't work. None of them worked for me for longer than a week or two.

"By the way, you skipped the *P* in SAPS. Did you forget one?"

"It looks like I got them a little out of order. Maybe I was just seeing if you were paying attention." They both laughed.

"Let's get the *P* on the board." David erased the last statement on the board and then wrote, "Rely upon external protection" He then rewrote, "Substitute another thought or action," beneath this.

"Now that we have that straightened out, let's talk about protection. Have you put filters on your computer, put your computer in a public place, or even cut off your Internet access to try to quit viewing?"

Jason thought about the many filters he had tried and bypassed and how he had moved the computer. It seemed to work temporarily, but the computer was easy to move somewhere else; even when it was placed in a high-traffic area, no one stayed up as late as he did when he wanted to view.

"I've tried many ways to protect myself from Internet pornography—all of the ones you mentioned plus some others."

"How have they worked out for you?" David asked.

Jason gave a half smile. He didn't like recalling the memory of failing at so many things, but this question was similar to a question from a previous session that imitated Dr. Phil's phrasing, "Not so well."

"Sometimes the protections can provide temporary relief from viewing, but they also mask dealing with the temptation. There are almost always some ways around the protections. In fact, some people go on binges when they travel, watching a lot of porn as they let loose the pent-up temptations that they haven't dealt with. These binges bring back all the negative consequences that they were trying to forsake.

"Others find ingenious ways to overcome the protections they set up, such as using work computers or friends' computers, buying their own private laptop, or asking a neighbor to use the wireless connection while theirs is 'temporarily down.' My clients have told me many excuses they've given for needing to borrow someone else's computer, or they use it when that person is away.

"Many of my recent clients used their smartphones or tablet computers to do their viewing. I was surprised to hear that many public libraries are sources for viewing pornography. With all the kids who access library computers, I thought they would have filters, but many libraries are foregoing or even removing filters to avoid the appearance of censorship; those are wrongly placed concerns in this instance, if you ask me. My guess is that as new types of protection arise, new ways to thwart them will arise as well."

"Are you saying that I should remove the Internet filters from my computer?" Jason asked incredulously.

"No." David smiled. "I'm not asking anything like that. I think the protections are important for our families, especially our children, and any others who may be using our electronics. We don't want to risk exposing others to pornography on our computers, phones, or televisions.

"In fact, when you're offered free movie channels that regularly feature pornography as part of a cable or satellite promotion, turn them down. You're not the only one who accesses your computers or televisions.

"The point is that the protections will not work for you because they don't deal with the temptation directly. You'll find ways around them or alternatives to satisfy the lingering temptation. When you start relying upon suppression, avoidance, protections, or substitution, the temptation hasn't been dealt with and will eventually win.

"Do you have any questions about how suppression, avoidance, protections, and substitution all prevent you from living a loving life?"

Before Jason could answer, David continued, "This concept is often the opposite of what many people believe before they start the program. We give a lot of power away, and the big four power takers, along with resisting, are the common ways we do so."

Jason paused and then replied, "You're right. The concepts are brand new to me. I thought that the only way to deal with the temptations was to avoid them. I've also substituted and tried protections as well, and I've discovered firsthand that they don't work."

"I like to use the acronym SAPS to help me remember and recognize that suppression, avoidance, protection, and substitution don't work because they don't effectively deal with the temptation. I like to think that the use of these methods saps one's power. Maybe this acronym will help you remember to deal with the temptation and to not suppress, avoid, protect, or substitute something else for it.

"We're almost done." David turned to the board and wrote, "Do it for yourself."

"Others in your life will naturally benefit when you succeed at living a loving life, but viewers experience the most success when they make these changes for their own benefit, not for others' benefit, even those closest to them. If they seek to do this to satisfy or provide benefits for someone else, their chances for success go down. For long-lasting change, you need to do it for yourself.

"As you recall, when we talked about your vision statement, I mentioned the importance of the benefits of your vision being for you, not for others. You made a minor tweak in your vision statement that made it more for you than for your family. No matter how altruistic you try to be, especially with your family, when you try to overcome such powerful addictions like viewing and doing, you need to do it for yourself.

"We're out of time but let's go over your homework."

Homework for Giving Away Your Power with SAPS:

1. Write your vision and read it to yourself five times. Modify it if necessary.
2. Write down the way you have used SAPS (suppression, avoidance, protections, and substitution) to avoid dealing with the urges to view. Note why each one of them does not work.
3. Read the AACV card for every viewing/doing or related temptation.
4. Continue using "choose" instead of "must," "have to," or any other language designed to compel.
5. It's time to remind yourself of the consequences of viewing and doing. Write your top five negatives and positives and state them (out loud if possible) while you write them.

Whiteboard Chapter 11

Take Responsibility for our choices and actions.

Tried and true failure paths—the power takers:

- Suppress the temptation.
- Avoid triggers and temptations.
- Rely upon external protection.
- Substitute another thought or action.

Do it for yourself.

CHAPTER 12:

Why Do We View Pornography?

When Jason arrived at David's home for their next session, he felt stressed for several reasons. He felt guilty for leaving the office early despite having a very productive day. He felt guilty that Becky didn't know he was coming here. He felt like he needed to be home with his kids. Not to mention he had the increased pressure of tax-filing deadlines at the end of the week.

In the past, during times like these, he felt viewing pornography would provide some stress relief. He had a clearer view of the consequences of his pornography viewing now and a vision to choose as an alternative. He also practiced embracing the stress to grow beyond his current comfort zone. But embracing it or not, he still felt the stress of his current circumstances.

After exchanging greetings, David suggested that they get right to work. "We're going to talk about why we view pornography and about some of the rationalizations that we've used in the past to justify our use. We started talking about some of these reasons last time. Let's dive a little deeper today.

"But before we start, how many times per day have you seen your vision in your mind since you were last here?"

Jason thought for a moment and answered, "Probably one or two times per day."

"Seeing it one or two times per day is good and will work well once you're into the maintenance phase of the program, but three to four would be the proper amount right now. When your vision becomes your focus, your power over pornography increases tremendously. Tonight, to help make your vision more real, find a picture that depicts your vision. You might find it in family photographs, in a magazine, or on the Internet. Once you have the picture, print it and display it in a place where you'll see it every day. Some people like to post it on their bathroom mirror."

"OK," Jason responded. "I think the more I focus on the vision, the greater my chances of achieving it. I like the bathroom mirror idea. I think I'll also find a picture to put near my computer at home."

"Great. Moving on, let's make a list." David turned to the familiar whiteboard and wrote, "Reasons why." He asked, "Why do you think you viewed pornography in the past?"

Jason had been thinking about this since the last session, and he had come up with some stronger reasons. "I believe that my sex drive is much stronger than my wife's. When she turns me down or I feel too distant from her, I need another outlet for my sex drive."

David listed "strong sex drive" and "need more than spouse provides."

"OK. What else?"

"When I see a beautiful woman in person or on TV, I'll sometimes get aroused and desire to view pornography."

David added "beautiful woman trigger" to the list.

"As we discussed last time, I've often turned to pornography as a stress reliever. When I feel stressed out, I'll sometimes view pornography to try to escape. I know it doesn't work, based on our last discussion, but it's been a primary reason for viewing in the past."

David added "relieve stress," "feel pleasure," and "get relief" to the list.

Jason continued. "Sometimes I just feel like I need it. I can't go to sleep without viewing—I can't relax. Other reasons that come to mind are the ones we covered last time, like feelings of boredom, anger, depression and sadness, or just feeling numb."

David wrote "need it," "relieve boredom," "outlet for anger," "help for depression," "help for sadness," and "try to stop feeling numb." The list on the whiteboard now consisted of the following items under "Reasons why:" *Strong sex drive, need more than spouse gives, beautiful woman trigger, relieve stress, feel pleasure, get relief, need it, relax, relieve boredom, outlet for anger, help for depression, help for sadness and try to stop feeling numb.*

Then he crossed out "Reasons why" and replaced it with "Rationalizations." David explained, "One of the requirements for overcoming pornography is to make sure we're telling the truth about our viewing. The reasons you just listed for viewing pornography are commonly listed by others, but they are still rationalizations. Another word for rationalization is lie."

Jason was a little stunned by David referring to his well-thought-out reasons as lies. David sensed Jason's surprise and suggested, "Let's dive deeper into why these are lies."

"One method I like to use to combat my tendency to rationalize is weighing the costs of the result to determine if the rationalization has any truth to it. For example, if I rationalize viewing because I have a strong sex drive, I'm saying that the satisfaction of my sex drive is more important than the consequences of viewing. What do you think?"

"When you put it that way I agree. The act of choosing consequences helps me recognize it more than before. Also, researching negative consequences helped me see the high cost of viewing and doing more directly than before. In other words, I think it helped me add the appropriate weight to the costs of viewing."

"Great. Let's move on. The biggest lie may be that relief equals happiness. We've already clarified the consequences of viewing pornography and identified that viewing in order to relieve stress actually results in more stress. Therefore, when you view pornography to attain relief, the relief comes at a high cost: killing what is most important to you. Viewed in this light, it's clear that not only is temporary relief not happiness, it is the opposite: misery. Do you agree?"

"I hadn't thought about it this way before beginning POP, but now I believe it wholeheartedly because I've experienced it. The relief comes at a very high price that is not worth paying."

"Let's go through a few of the other items on the list to illustrate. Let's start with the strong sex drive. I don't know the exact science, but I believe it's more or less a fact that men have a stronger sex drive than women, with some exceptions of course. When we rationalize that this justifies viewing pornography, we say that our strong sex drive has to be satisfied at the cost of our self-confidence, ability to love, ability to have meaningful relationships, success on the job, and happiness.

"Worth it or not?"

"Not."

David crossed through the words "strong sex drive."

"Not getting as much sex from our spouse as we desire seems similar to a strong sex drive. When we satisfy our perceived need for more sex than we can get from our spouse by viewing and doing, we in essence say, 'Because I'm not having sex frequently enough, I'm going to take action that will shrink the love in my most important relationships, deaden my career, and...' you can fill in the blanks with some of the negative consequences you discovered in your research that matter most to you.

"Doesn't make much sense, does it?" David asked.

"You're right. Put in that light, it doesn't make much sense at all."

"Worth it or not?"

"Not."

He crossed it off.

"The beautiful woman trigger. To see a beautiful woman and rationalize looking at pornography is to punish ourselves and deny our right to choose our reaction." He crossed it off.

David continued. "Relieve stress. This is my favorite. Just to review, in the past when you sought to relieve stress by viewing pornography, how did you feel?"

"I felt some temporary relief followed by increased stress."

"How long did the temporary relief last?"

Jason softly said, "Less than a minute."

"How and what do you feel after that time is up?"

As Jason reflected on the feelings of guilt, shame, and low self-worth, he replied, "Worse than before viewing and doing."

"'Worse' is a very nonspecific word. My guess is that it includes all the items from your list of top five negative consequences. Am I right?"

"I guess so."

"Do you have any other ways to describe the feeling without delving into the specifics?"

Jason didn't understand at first, but he started thinking about it, and the word "stress" popped into his mind. As soon as he thought it, he blurted it out to David.

David smiled. "How cloudy do our consequences need to be for us to seek relief from stress by doing something that only adds to it?"

Jason had to repeat the question in his mind to get the full impact.

David continued, "As you mentioned, the relief from stress is very temporary, and then the stress itself is magnified. Can you describe that process more clearly?"

Jason quickly responded, "When I compound experiencing the consequences of viewing pornography on top of the stress I'm already feeling, it magnifies the stress."

David smiled. "In fact, as we discussed, it can lead to a cycle of stress. Once the consequences of the viewing incident add to the stress, then a viewer feels the need to react to the stress and try to relieve it by viewing and doing. This only adds more to the stress, and the downward cycle continues.

"I think the same can be said for seeking relief from other negative emotions. One of the consequences of viewing pornography that you clarified was a lack of love, which can easily be interpreted as sadness. The response to the added sadness is more viewing, which leads to more sadness, and the downward cycle continues on and on.

"I hope you can see that whenever we try to rationalize viewing pornography, we're only lying to ourselves and preventing our realization of the benefits of living a loving life." David proceeded to cross off the remaining items on the list.

Jason nodded in silent agreement.

"Now that I've explained how our rationalizations are lies, let me provide a new list of feelings, and you can tell me if you've experienced any of these feelings over the past forty-eight hours." David wrote a new list on the board that included the following words: irritated, deprived, denied, angry, sad, anxious, fearful, nervous, worried, stressed, bored, and aroused.

As Jason scanned the list, he said, "I know I've been feeling a little bit of fear. I've failed so many times in the past that, although my confidence is growing with each temptation I deal with, I'm afraid that I will fail again."

David nodded, prompting Jason to continue.

"I feel deprived when I think that I may never view again. But success in the program means never viewing again, and I still have the desire to view pornography. This makes me feel like I am denying myself, but I think that's normal when you're trying to quit.

"I've also felt anxious and nervous. I'm used to viewing pornography almost every night or whenever I want to. Now that I'm not, I feel anxious."

David was listening closely. "Let's address some of these feelings. If they are left to fester and not dealt with directly, they can block your success.

"You've defined yourself as a pornography viewer. It's now embedded on your self-image. Changing that image can be scary. Whenever we seek to change our self-image, we're redefining who we are, and we feel fear, anxiety, and discomfort.

"These feelings will probably last another two or three days before they shrink and dissipate as your comfort zone expands over the next few weeks. I picked up a book a few years ago titled *Feel the Fear and Do It Anyway*. I think that is a great motto to live by. Whenever we venture out of our comfort zone, especially when we try to change our definition of ourselves, we will feel fear. The realization that this is a short-term feeling should provide you with assurance that you're on the right track.

"The power of your vision and the clarity of the consequences will give you the strength to power through feelings of fear and anxiety. Do you feel that it's worth feeling fear, anxiety, and discomfort for a short period of time to be able to live a loving life?"

Jason answered, "I think it's worth it, but what do you mean by short period of time? If I imagine experiencing fear and anxiety for several months, I'm not so sure. I don't have the confidence that I can live with the discomfort for that long without reverting back to viewing."

"Let me clarify," David began. "I didn't explain the length of time you can expect these feelings. The fear, anxiety, and discomfort are only temporary. You'll feel less of them today than you did yesterday, and then each following day, you'll feel less of them as your comfort zone expands and your power increases.

"I expect you'll be free of these feelings in about three weeks, and they'll begin diminishing well before then. Now that you have a better idea of the time frame, do you feel that these temporary feelings are worth the positive consequences?"

Jason responded, "Now that you've explained it, I think it's absolutely worth it. However, I still don't understand how these feelings diminish so quickly."

"As you continue to exercise your power of choice and embrace the discomfort, you'll experience firsthand how quickly the feelings diminish. Your comfort zone expands at a brisk pace.

"I hope you'll also be willing to believe that you don't need to prove yourself right about failing. One of the prerequisites for success is to believe that you will be successful. Because you've failed in the past, you may not have the firm belief in success that you would like. I sense that as you're learning and understanding the concepts we're discussing, your confidence in yourself is increasing. I also sense that you are truly starting to believe that you'll succeed. Am I right?"

"Yeah. My perspective is changing, and I'm growing more confident that I can do this."

"Good. Let's tackle some of the other thoughts and feelings.

"I'm glad you mentioned feeling deprived. It is one of the most common obstacles to success, and it requires repetition in order to combat. One of the essential elements of this program is the freedom of choice. We've already discussed how you exercise your freedom to choose any time you face an urge or temptation.

"Remember, one of the failure paths is to believe that we only make the decision once, and it applies to all future decision points. The thought process that follows this perspective leads to feelings of deprivation and denial. When you believe you will no longer ever be able to view and do, you naturally feel deprived.

"The solution is to continue to change the perspective and the process. In the future, when you decide to choose to live a loving life or to view pornography, you're choosing that action for that instance only. You can choose differently the next instance.

"When you're free to choose to view pornography at any time, do you feel deprived?"

"No," Jason responded. "How can you feel deprived when you know you can view anytime you want?"

"Exactly. Let's explore this a little more.

"We've discovered that when you make a decision that lasts forever, you are using a form of force, compelling yourself to make the same decision tomorrow that you made today. I know this is review, but the repetition is important. How do we typically act when we feel forced to do something?"

"I tend to rebel against it, even if I don't say anything."

"Right. We tend to rebel against actions that attempt to force us to do something. We've spent time in a past session on using force language against ourselves, so we won't dwell on it now.

"Some say that this contradicts the power of commitment, but you'll find that choosing in every instance empowers you and takes away feelings of deprivation or denial.

"Sometimes we have to tell ourselves that no one and no circumstances can take away our freedom to choose. If we don't remind our whiny viewer-doer mind that we always have a choice, we will feel like a victim and enter into the cycle that leads to relapse.

"How can you feel deprived knowing that you can always choose to view and do? The choice is always up to you.

"Let me explain it a little differently. When you realize you have the choice, you realize you're not depriving yourself at all; you're choosing to live a loving life this time, knowing that you can choose differently any time you want."

Jason understood most of what David explained. Until starting POP, he attributed his relapses to his lack of self-discipline. Now he felt that overcoming the addiction may not be about self-discipline at all, but instead has everything to do with the freedom to choose. "Knowing that I can view pornography anytime I want feels more powerful than telling myself I must have the self-discipline to never view again."

David's eyes brightened. "I see that you used the words 'must' and 'self-discipline' in the same sentence. I think that calls for a MuHa laugh." David did his best impression of an evil-sounding MuHa laugh. Jason chuckled, thinking, *David is not very convincing when he tries to sound evil.*

David continued. "The laugh is not only for the MuHa lie but also for the self-discipline lie. Like you, many people believe the reason for their viewing addiction is due to their own lack of self-discipline. As we've discussed, it's not about self-discipline but about choice.

"Let's go back to the power of choosing for just the current instance. One of the sayings I picked up from twelve-step meetings was 'one day at a time.' The choice doesn't seem so daunting if we just choose for today, knowing we can choose differently tomorrow. If we just live a loving life today, we'll deal with tomorrow when it comes. There is power to staying in the present instead of worrying about the future.

"I've modified the saying to fit my needs: 'one instance at a time.' We can choose differently every time we're faced with the choice. We don't have to choose for a whole day but just for this instance.

"So, the next time you're feeling denied or deprived, tell yourself that you can choose to view any time you want to. Your choice to live a loving life and to experience your vision is for this instance only.

"The concept of free choice for this instance only is crucial to your success, so we continued to emphasize it in today's session. I can tell you're tired, so let's call it a night. You are now armed with the heart of the program, but you're not quite finished. There are a few important concepts and practices we need to cover as you continue taking your power back from viewing and doing.

"Don't forget to do your homework. The main reason for the homework is not only to make sure you understand the concepts but also to help them become a part of you. The homework helps prevent the clouds from coming back to your vision and to your list of negative and positive consequences."

Homework for Why Do We View Pornography:

1. Write down the three top reasons you've used in the past to justify viewing. Write down why they are lies.
2. Write down the feelings you have before you view and how these feelings change or are amplified after viewing.
3. Write down the following: "I'm choosing for this instance only. I always have the right to choose differently." Repeat it five times.

Whiteboard Chapter 12-1

Reasons Why:
- Strong sex drive
- Need more than spouse gives
- Beautiful woman trigger
- Relieve stress
- Feel pleasure
- Relax
- Get relief
- Need it
- Relieve boredom
- Outlet for anger
- Help for depression
- Help for sadness
- Try to stop feeling numb

Whiteboard Chapter 12-2

Reasons why: Rationalizations:
- Strong sex drive
- Need more than spouse provides
- Beautiful woman trigger
- Relieve stress
- Relax
- Feel pleasure
- Get relief
- Need it
- Relieve boredom
- Outlet for anger
- Help for depression
- Help for sadness
- Try to stop feeling numb

Whiteboard Chapter 12-3

Facing Temporary Feelings:
- Irritated
- Deprived
- Denied
- Angry
- Sad
- Anxious
- Fearful
- Nervous
- Worried
- Stressed
- Bored
- Aroused

Note: *Please refer to poweroverpornography.com/rationalizations to review a current list of rationalizations of viewers. Please add some of yours to the list.*

CHAPTER 13:

Repairing the Damage to Yourself

Jason walked briskly to David's door. He enjoyed his sessions with David and was eager to start the next one.

"Jason, I haven't asked specific questions about the genesis of your addiction, and I don't know how long you've struggled with it. But I've seen that no matter the reasons someone started viewing or how long he or she has been viewing, the viewer's self-esteem and confidence are damaged. Viewers see a part of their true selves as failures.

"Most viewers recognize this, but I've worked with some who adamantly deny that their viewing has changed them, damaged their self-esteem, or lessened their capacity to love. Only after they experience the power of the program do they realize how damaged they were.

"Now that you know how to live a loving life and have begun to do so, the negative emotions and feelings that emanate from a damaged self-image should diminish. I think you'll be pleased with the next part of the formula; it speeds the process of reducing the negative and increasing the positive."

"I'm glad you mentioned that my confidence is growing. The changes are subtle. I don't really notice them until I compare my confidence level now with my confidence level before meeting with you. I believe the increase in confidence and self-esteem is real, but so far the changes are small.

"I also have the experience of the six months of pornography sobriety after I completed the twelve-step program. During that relatively happy time, I realized that my self-image and important relationships all suffered while I was a viewer.

"But I'm a bit puzzled by your comment about perceiving part of one's true self as a failure."

"I haven't encountered any viewer who, deep-down, didn't consider him- or herself a failure. Almost all viewers first try to stop in conventional ways, such as exercising self-discipline, installing filters on their computer, keeping their computer in a common area, and so on. They may experience abstinence for a few days, weeks, or months, but they end up going back to viewing, thus failing in their attempts to stop.

"The failures continue in a cycle, and they take their toll by increasing shame and guilt while stealing self-esteem, confidence, and value. The failure cycle eventually causes viewers to see themselves as failures because they don't have the power to stop viewing by themselves.

"When a viewer tries a twelve-step program and experiences initial success and confidence and then relapses, it can be a tough blow to that person's confidence; it can cause him or her to feel like a failure. They think, *If I can't even succeed at a program that is successful for others, there must be no hope for me.*

"This is another lie that I want to help viewers confront so they can move forward in exercising their free choice to choose a loving life.

"Sometimes viewers rationalize that viewing is OK, and they have many reasons to do it, from 'my sex drive is stronger than my wife's' to 'I'm not hurting anyone' to 'it's natural' and 'everyone does it.' We've already discussed these lies. They don't help overcome the failure syndrome.

"Every viewer I've met realizes—some with strong knowledge and some only deep in his or her heart—that viewing is wrong and that the failure to stop is just that, a failure. It defines who they are. As they try to compartmentalize the failure to viewing, it bleeds into every other aspect of their lives, damaging relationships, hurting work performance, and bringing all the other negative consequences you discovered in your research.

"With this background on the failure syndrome, let me get to the heart of the answer to your question about true self.

"I believe you came into this world as a strong, confident human being with divine attributes. But through your viewing and potentially through other effects of your upbringing, you lost a part of your true self. The strength and confidence were replaced with failure, shame, and selfishness, while the divine attributes drifted to the far reaches of your mind and heart.

"Does this answer your question?"

Jason was touched. Before he met David, he had believed he was not capable of recovery. He recalled how dejected he was when he returned to the twelve-step meeting just the previous month. He now felt hope that he could live a loving life. "Yeah, you answered it well."

"Let's turn to the supercharger of confidence, self-esteem, and true self. Have you heard of affirmations?"

"I know what the word means in general, but I am not sure what you mean."

"Affirmations are beliefs about who you want to become. When you recite them, you repeat attributes that you desire but may not have. In essence, you state your desired attributes as if they are already a part of you.

"You tell your subconscious that you are the type of person you say you are. Your subconscious then works to make these affirmations come true.

"I generally don't believe in quick fixes or gimmicky answers to hard problems, but I've found that affirmations can build a firm path of success for viewers. I think the inherent consequences of viewing, such as shame, guilt, self-loathing, and the inability to love deeply become imbedded into the self-image of the viewer.

"The best way to begin ridding yourself of this negative self-image is to live a loving life. I wish I could tell you that your self-image would change immediately, but I've found that it's a slow change. One of the ways to help your self-image change a little more quickly is to use affirmations. Your self-image impacts all areas of your life, so we want to do everything we can to change it quickly. Does that make sense?"

"I think so, but I'm not really sure what the affirmations are and how I go about using them to heal my damaged self-image."

"The best way to explain affirmations more specifically may be through example. Here are some." David began writing as he spoke. Seeing them on the whiteboard gave Jason a chance to dwell on each example and to see which ones resonated with him.

- I am a child of God.
- I like myself.
- I possess divine attributes.
- I am free to choose at all times.
- I feel calm and peaceful.
- The worth of my soul is infinite.
- I enjoy new experiences.
- I am a loving person.
- I welcome the discomfort that accompanies positive change.
- I am worthy of being loved.
- I feel terrific.
- I have strong relationships with my wife and children.
- I forgive myself.
- I build people up.
- Each action I take is my choice and my responsibility.
- I have an excellent career.
- I am prosperous.
- I am grateful.
- I love my family deeply.

"I know this violates my rule of five, but I think you get the gist of what affirmations are. Do you have any you would like to add, change, or take off the list? Don't be too eager to remove them. You'll have a chance to narrow the list to the ones that are most important to you in a minute."

"Perhaps we could add one to the list about healthy living. I haven't always taken the best care of my health but feel that it's an important part of self-esteem, at least for me."

"Oh, I also think my role as a father deserves to be separate from my role as a husband. They're the two relationships I value most, so why don't we separate them?

"No problem. This is your list, so we want to make it real for you. I've simply started the list to give you some choices and help you see what an affirmation is."

David added, "I live a healthy lifestyle," "I am a good husband," and "I am a good father," to the list.

"The next step in your program is to select the five most meaningful affirmations and recite them to yourself once per day. The rule of five applies, but your list of five affirmations is not permanent. You may want to change them as your challenges change and you change.

"Please review the list and select the five affirmations you most want. This will be your homework. We don't always follow up on your home-work, but we'll plan to follow up on this one.

"There's one other thing I want to mention before you leave. Some self-esteem gurus would have you believe that daily affirmations are the end-all and be-all in improving your self-image. In truth, neglect-ing other aspects of building strong self-esteem will impede your prog-ress despite using daily affirmations. We know there are many aspects of good self-esteem that are important, the primary one being living a loving life. The other major aspects include the following."

David spoke as he wrote them on the board. "Set and achieve worthy goals, live your life congruently with your values, feel gratitude on a daily basis, spend time with those you love, be present by focusing on the per-son or task at hand, and serve others."

"We won't get into a lot of these vital aspects of building your self-esteem, but please know that they're important and use them in your life. One thing to keep in mind concerning living congruently with your values is to make sure your values are consistent with true and proven principles. Adopting values that are not in line with the truth will result in low self-esteem and limit your chances of happiness.

"Affirmations work. They help you change your thought patterns and begin building the self-image of someone living a loving life. They are simple to implement. They also begin increasing your self-esteem in a short period of time."

Homework for Repairing the Damage to Yourself:

1. Select and write down the five top affirmations that you will recite to yourself every day.
2. Select the same time of day to recite them, and repeat them every day.
3. Continue reciting the AACV card with every instance of temptation. It's vital to do this without exception every time you experience a temptation.
4. Review the following list of other long-term self-esteem builders and make a general plan to implement them.
   a. Set and achieve worthy goals
   b. Live your life congruently with your values
   c. Feel gratitude on a daily basis
   d. Spend deliberate, focused time with those you love
   e. Be present by focusing on the person or task at hand.
   f. Serve others.
   g. Base your values on true and proven principles.

Whiteboard Chapter 13-1

Affirmations

- I am a child of God.
- I like myself.
- I possess divine attributes.
- I am free to choose at all times.
- I feel calm and peaceful.
- The worth of my soul is infinite.
- I am a loving person.
- I welcome the feeling of discomfort that accompanies positive change.
- I am worthy of being loved.
- I feel terrific.
- I have strong relationships with my wife and children.
- I forgive myself.
- I build people up.
- Each action I take is my choice and my responsibility.
- I have an excellent career.
- I am prosperous.
- I am grateful.
- I love my family deeply.
- I live a healthy lifestyle.
- I am a good husband.
- I am a good father.

Whiteboard Chapter 13-2

Essential Self-Esteem Builders:

- Set and achieve worthy goals
- Live your life congruently with your values
- Feel gratitude on a daily basis
- Spend time with those you love
- Be present by focusing on the person or task at hand
- Serve others

Note: *Please refer to* poweroverpornography.com/affirmations *to review a larger list of affirmations. Choose those most impactful to you. Please share some of your affirmations as well.*

Chapter 14:

Repairing Your Relationships

Jason woke up early the next Saturday morning. This was usually the day he slept in, but he had refined his list of affirmations the previous night and still had "good husband" and "good father" on his mind. He decided to make breakfast.

Bailey usually awoke before Jason did. He smiled at the thought of her bouncing on the bed to wake them up most Saturday mornings. She would be surprised to see him already awake.

As he tiptoed to the kitchen, he heard Bailey's door open. She was running toward his bedroom and was startled when she ran right into him. "Daddy? Where are you going?" She seemed worried that he was leaving.

Jason picked her up and hugged her. "I'm going with you to the kitchen. Do you want to help me make breakfast?"

Bailey was too excited to speak. She nodded her head, and most of the rest of her body followed in an exaggerated motion.

While Jason looked in the cupboards to get pancake flour, Bailey looked out the window. "Dad, I see a turtle."

Jason would normally continue looking for items and utter something like, "That's nice," but this time he looked out the window with Bailey and asked "Where?"

"Right there, in the big cloud on top of the sky, silly."

Jason took Bailey outside. They identified cloud shapes for thirty minutes, sometimes sitting, sometimes laying on their backs. He couldn't remember laughing so much with Bailey in a long time. They especially laughed hard when she asked what a Scooby Doo was and Jason tried to explain.

As their next session started, David stared directly into Jason's eyes, and asked, "Well?"

Jason knew he was referring to the homework, so he opened his notebook to show David his top five affirmations.

I am a child of God.
I am free to choose at all times.
I have an excellent career.
I live a healthy lifestyle.
I am a good husband.
I am a good father.

Before David could say anything about the list, Jason defended it. "I know there are six items, not five, but I wasn't willing to give up any of the six."

David nodded in agreement. "The rule of five is designed to help you focus and to make you think about your highest priorities. I can tell that you put some thought into this list, so the rule accomplished that objective. I also don't see a problem to having six affirmations instead of five.

"I like to use the rule of five on affirmation lists so that reciting the list is a quick exercise that can fit into anyone's day. After you recite it a few times, you're able to memorize it so that you can still recite it even if you misplace the list.

"I think your six items fit the spirit of the rule. The big question is, do they resonate with you, and when you recite them, do you feel your self-esteem and general well-being increase?"

Jason responded, "I think so. I kept thinking about your statement that the list is not permanent, so I plan to keep referring back to the longer list to make changes periodically. But right now, the list feels good to me.

"I have to admit that I thought it was a bit silly at first to recite these statements but I always smile and feel good after I do it, so I think it actually may help. I noticed that they are all phrased in present tense and are statements of being for the most part instead of want-to-be statements. I think there's something to that."

David smiled. "The affirmations have less impact if they're phrased as goals or want-to-be statements. Your viewing and doing have negatively changed your self-image and self-esteem at the brain level. We need to convince the subconscious part of your brain that you are healing so that it does not revert back to the self-image of the viewer and doer who feels like a failure.

"When I first encountered affirmations as a way to improve my life, I had the same reaction that you did. I wondered what good it would do for me to say the same things to myself every day. But I'm glad I didn't let my inner skeptic win. It's made a tremendous difference in my life in more ways than just correcting the damage from viewing and doing.

"I was able to change my self-image to one of a confident, loving person more quickly than I could have otherwise. I'm glad you've relaxed your inner skeptic as well so that you can feel the power and the healing that comes with reciting daily affirmations.

"I encourage you to recite them every day, and don't forget to refine and change them periodically. I hope you find them as powerful in your life as I've found them in mine.

"Your self-image and self-esteem power your attitude, achievement, and ability to care for yourself and others. We did not spend much time going over the other long-term self-esteem builders, but please take them seriously and make them part of your everyday life. As you do so, your self-image will change and your self-esteem will grow.

"If we expanded our discussion of the self-esteem builders to the level they deserve, then our POP program would become a self-esteem program. We'll save that for another day," David said with a chuckle. "Today, we're going to focus on some simple things you can do to repair your relationship with Becky.

"Speaking of full programs, there are entire courses on relationship building, but for now, I want to provide you with some simple steps to help rebuild your relationship with your spouse. These tips are not the whole solution, but they are a start.

"Before we discuss rebuilding your relationship, let's talk about temptations. Are you experiencing the same number of temptations per day now versus when you first started the AACV process?"

"No, I'm still experiencing temptations to view and do, but I am only tempted one or two times per day now. Some days I'm not tempted at all. It seems like I'm making progress."

Jason was surprised that David didn't greet his answer with more enthusiasm.

"That is what I suspected may be happening," David said matter-of-factly. "You may not be practiced enough to thrive with only one or no temptations per day. This process takes practice, and I think you may need more."

"What do you mean? I am dealing with each temptation as it comes using the AACV card. I thought it was a good thing to have fewer temptations per day."

"I think you need more temptations per day so you can practice. We'll talk about it in the next module, but practice is what keeps us sharp and helps us make new feelings of SAD (stress, anxiety, and discomfort) into positive automatic reactions. It takes a lot of practice to master anything, including living a life of love."

"You don't think I should make up temptations for myself do you?" Jason asked dismissively.

"That's exactly what I would like you to do. For now, you need practice dealing with temptations at least two to three times per day. I know it seems counterintuitive to create thoughts that mimic temptations, but if you don't get enough practice, relapse becomes more likely."

"It seems a little strange to me, but so have other parts of the course at first. And they worked like magic. I'll continue to trust in the program and create temptations to ensure I'm practicing the AACV process at least two to three times per day. I'm not sure I'll be able to keep creating them every day forever though. It seems like it could get tedious."

"The purpose of creating your own temptation-mimicking thoughts is to practice acknowledging and accepting them, exercising your power to choose, and then choosing your vision. Make sure you immediately start the AACV process once you create a temptation. Each time you do, your practice makes it easier and more automatic to use the same process for each future temptation.

"By the way, I've stated both 'create a thought that mimics a temptation' and 'create a temptation.' Let me explain the difference. I believe that some temptations originate external to each of us and some originate within us. So, I like to think that the phrases 'creating a temptation' and 'creating a thought that mimics a temptation' are both valid and, although slightly different, can be interchangeable. Just recognize that the result is the same--they both initiate practice dealing with temptation.

"You won't need to create thoughts that mimic temptations every day forever. It's just for the next few weeks. We'll get into the why and how of long-term practice in the next session. I think you'll like the low-maintenance nature of the long-term practice.

"Now, let's finally get back to relationships.

"When someone's relationship with his or her spouse is truly in tatters, I recommend professional counseling. What we'll cover next is not comprehensive and not designed for repairing deeply troubled relationships. I don't get the sense that your relationship with Becky is in deep trouble, but only you and she can tell for sure. As you assess your relationship with your wife and as she provides you feedback about it, please seek professional counseling if you feel it will help.

"One of the common responses I hear when we teach this module is: 'our relationship is fine; it doesn't need rebuilding.'

"In your case, you've discussed with me that you realize the drifting apart that you and Becky have experienced is due to your viewing. Realization is the first step to taking responsibility so you can begin to make changes. This is a big first step, and you should feel good that you've already taken it.

"You've already made the biggest change toward helping your relationship with your wife by starting on the path to living a loving life. When you are no longer a viewer and doer, you become transformed; you become more capable of loving; you are better able to see your wife's beauty, and you have a greater desire to love her.

"Transformed may be too strong of a word, but I think it is appropriate. Let me explain. Often, the changes in the love and emotions you feel toward your spouse happen gradually. Sometimes viewers don't notice the negative feelings caused by viewing until they look back over a several-month time period to see the lack of love in their lives and the negative feelings directed toward their spouse.

"Once they see the contrast of their viewing life versus their loving life, they notice the transformation. Once you see the transformation, it's easier to recognize that small changes to your relationship skills don't amount to much without the changes to you and your viewing and the inside-out transformation that the POP program brings.

"Now that you are beginning to experience living a loving life, let's discuss ways you can increase the pace of rebuilding your relationships in other ways. We'll focus on physical and emotional intimacy.

"It is vital to reclaim intimacy if you want to rebuild your relationship with your wife. When you are a viewer, you build a false intimacy with pornography and its images. This false intimacy prevents you from feeling real intimacy with your spouse.

"It takes effort to reestablish real intimacy. I've found that there are steps you can take to reestablish it more quickly and on a solid foundation. Let me cover some of those steps with you next."

David began writing as he spoke, "As Patrick Carnes said, 'True intimacy is formed over years of trust, respect, kindness, affection.' He also noted that intimacy is an integral part of your recovery."[iii]

"The key is to develop a new, healthy model of intimacy that incorporates more than the physical. This is something that you can't do alone; you need to involve your spouse. Speaking of involving your spouse, let's pause and discuss a difficult but important part of repairing your relationship.

"As you know, the initial portion of POP is designed to work without spousal involvement. However, this is not a permanent part of POP and I want to tell you why. Scientific comparisons of the success of pornography addiction treatment programs, mostly twelve-step programs, show that there is greater and longer-lasting success when spouses are involved.

"When spouses are told about the problem and involved in the recovery, success rates are higher. POP users experience greater success in general but experience an increase in success rates when spouses are involved.

"The reason we don't involve spouses at the beginning of POP is that the fear of disclosure to a spouse keeps many viewers from seeking help. We want to help as many viewers as possible, so we haven't made spousal involvement an initial requirement of the program.

"I now want to revisit this with you for three reasons. I've just mentioned the first reason. Studies show greater success with disclosure in other treatment programs. You will see greater success in POP if you disclose your past viewing and doing to your spouse.

"The second reason is the ethical responsibility we have to our spouse to be transparent. If we're hiding something in our past, it may be difficult to connect on a deep level.

"Marriage and serious dating relationships depend upon honesty and trust. When we choose not to disclose our past viewing and doing, we're keeping secrets that fracture the honesty and trust. Often, the viewer's spouse blames him or herself for the rocky relationship and the absence of deep love. Correcting this perspective is the right thing to do.

"I like the way Mark Butler, a family therapist specializing in treating pornography addiction put it. He states that authenticity in a relationship is vital for the intimacy of the relationship.

"His research explains that 'withholding disclosure in a marriage relationship can bring about a fragmented relationship…When pair-bond partners relate through the remaining fragments of themselves—not willing to be fully, intimately known—or mask their authentic self behind false personas, the relationship becomes a stage façade of intimacy rather than a real-life enactment of intimacy.'[iv]

"The third reason is spiritual in nature. Disclosure results in quicker and more complete healing. Your disclosure to me and especially to the head of your congregation help, but repentance and the associated healing is incomplete without disclosing and apologizing to the person harmed by your actions. In this case, that person is Becky.

"The decision to disclose or not is up to you. I just wanted you to know some of the positive consequences that result from disclosure. Although the reactions of a spouse are hard to predict, the benefits of disclosure outweigh the potentially negative response in most cases. I also wanted you to know it's important, and I hope that you'll consider it in the future as you work on improving your relationship with Becky."

"OK," Jason answered nervously, "but I still don't know how she would react if I told her. I probably would have quit POP early if I thought a key part of it was involving her. I feel greater love for her, but I'll have to work up to disclosing my addiction to her."

David responded, "That is a common response. I just want you to keep an open mind to it. As I've said, part of reigniting the intimacy in your marriage is being honest with your spouse. When you're holding back a major part of your past that impacted her life and her relationship with you, it may be more difficult to rebuild your relationship.

"I want to see you succeed with POP, so consider sharing your past with Becky to enhance your chances. Revealing your own battles and vulnerabilities can bring you closer together. Will you consider it?"

"I understand how it can be helpful, but I still think I need some time to work up to it."

"OK. Let me know before you discuss it with her, and I can provide some tips that may help. Let's move on in our discussion of improving your intimate relationship with Becky.

"One of the keys in developing healthy intimacy is to create a joint vision of intimacy. That is, what do each of you and both of you want sexual intimacy to be like in your marriage?

"This means you need to discuss the kind of relationship, including the sexual relationship, you want to have as a couple. If you don't talk, you won't be able to experience true intimacy. Now, if you're like me, these can be difficult conversations, so here are some ways to start them.

"I often start conversations about intimacy with my wife by sincerely expressing my love to her and then saying something along the lines of, 'Intimacy is an important part of us feeling close to each other,' followed by asking, 'How do you feel we're doing as a couple with intimacy?'

"Once you open the conversation, continue asking questions like, 'What do you think we should change?' 'What can I do better?' 'What kind of sexual relationship do you desire and expect?'

"Just having this conversation with your spouse without an agenda and without the motive to make her feel guilty is a way of rebuilding your relationship. But don't be disappointed if it doesn't go as planned. The many years of low trust, respect, kindness, and affection often mean that some rebuilding time needs to happen before a conversation about intimacy goes well.

"An additional impediment to this conversation is the false sense of intimacy that viewing and doing gave you. It has been an escape from real-life intimacy, and it will take some time to turn around. So, how do you help this sort of conversation happen and produce true intimacy?" As David gave the following explanations, he also wrote them on the whiteboard.

"**Risk being the first to speak**. When you accept the risk of rejection and you reveal your internal struggles, you create trust and open up the ability to discuss joint problems. This is a big step that actually helps you heal. You can't maintain a viewer mind while revealing your deep thoughts. According to Patrick Carnes, 'In healthy relationships, intimacy becomes possible when people accept the risk of rejection and reveal their internal struggles.'[v]

"**Be a listener first and a talker second**. It's important that your focus be on the conversation. Your past viewing and doing makes you want to focus on almost anything but your spouse and the conversation. Choose to keep your focus on her. Listening fully is one of the great esteem and relationship builders and, therefore, a key to rebuilding real intimacy."

Jason agreed but was puzzled. "What do you mean when you say 'fully'? I think I'm a good listener, but maybe I need some help."

"You know you're fully listening when the only thoughts that come into your mind are pertinent to the conversation (or, if others do come to mind, you choose to refocus on listening), you are not putting together your response in your mind while your spouse is still talking, and you notice your spouse's emotions and body language in addition to his or her voice.

"There is a lot more to listening, but the three tips we just mentioned, (1) no other irrelevant thoughts while listening; (2) no forming your response while the other is talking; and (3) noticing emotions, body language, and tone of voice, will put you most of the way there.

"**Avoid becoming defensive**. Your viewer-doer mind will revert to the shame and guilt of the addiction, and the ensuing low self-esteem will want you to be defensive. When defensive thoughts come into your mind, choose to listen instead. Withdrawal is another defense mechanism, so watch for it and stay engaged.

"**Share**. The hiding mentality of the viewer and doer means you haven't practiced sharing as much. Begin sharing your thoughts and feelings more. Keeping them inside can inhibit intimacy. You may want to write down your thoughts and feelings during the day so that you can share them with your spouse later.

"**Be dependable, even for hard things**. A natural consequence of viewing and doing is to be less dependable and to avoid accepting or accomplishing difficult tasks. You'll naturally feel more dependable and willing to take on harder tasks as you start living a loving life. But trust starts with dependability, so emphasize this goal. Remember, there are few if any tasks or meetings that are a higher priority than your spouse and children.

"**Demonstrate your love**. Words are less powerful than actions. Plan date nights each week with Becky around what you know she likes to do. Think about little actions that will mean a lot to her. This will mean a great deal in showing your commitment, and it will lead to greater marital intimacy.

"**Be honest**. Honesty is a key to intimacy."

"When you approach reestablishing intimacy by engaging in conversations that use the six steps we just listed, you will be on the right path to rebuilding your relationship. The real intimacy that you'll start to feel will help you in your quest to live a loving life. It will make your physical intimacy more satisfying, and it will increase your overall well-being as an individual and as a spouse.

"You'll form greater trust in your relationship and have a sense of connection that will provide happiness and satisfaction. You'll also feel less emotional pain; you may even experience some relief from old emotional pain that stems from your upbringing, for example. You'll also feel your self-esteem and self-image grow.

"I'm sure you realize that this is just part of rebuilding your relationship with your spouse. The daily things you say and do will play a major role in rebuilding the trust, intimacy, and love that make your marriage the key relationship in your life and a major source of happiness and fulfillment.

"I hope you also realize that taking steps to improve your relationship will have a minor impact if you don't continue living a loving life. As harsh as it may sound, remember that you're just one view away from the viewer life filled with hatred, selfishness, anger, and misery."

Homework for Repairing Your Relationships:

1. Develop a plan to implement the six components of building intimacy into your relationship.
   a. Write each component. Write one action you'll take this week to implement that component in your life.
2. Have a conversation with your spouse about intimacy. Use the listening tips. Write down your summary of the conversation.
3. Don't let the consequences get cloudy. Write down your top five negatives and top five positives again.
4. Experience at least two to three temptations per day and follow the AACV card to deal with them. If you don't have this number of temptations come to you naturally, create additional thoughts that mimic temptations. You're still in need of practice.

Whiteboard Chapter 14

True intimacy is formed over years of trust, respect, kindness, and affection.

Intimacy is an integral part of your recovery. It is more than just physical.

Talk about it:

- Risk being the first to speak. Ask questions.
- Listen fully without becoming defensive.
- Share.
- Be dependable.
- Demonstrate your love. Actions speak louder than words.
- Be honest.

Note: *Please refer to* poweroverpornography.com/relationships *to review the latest tips on improving your most valued relationships. Please also share your success stories and learning experiences.*

CHAPTER 15:

Practice, the Power in Repetition

Jason felt hope as he left David's house. He sensed the power in the concepts David had taught him, and he was already practicing them with success.

Jason smiled as he looked forward to greeting and spending time with his family. With the relationship session fresh in his mind, he set a mental goal to make everyone in the family smile, laugh, and enjoy the evening.

Jason walked in the front door as quietly as he could. He wanted to surprise his family. As he crept into the family room, he heard the TV. He crouched down and crept behind the sofa. Then, he jumped up and shouted "Boo!"

Mike and Bailey both screamed. They were startled, and Mike was a little embarrassed about screaming like a girl. They both looked at Jason and in unison said, "Dad!" When they saw Jason's smile, they laughed. Bailey jumped over the back of the sofa and into Jason's arms. She hugged him tightly.

Becky heard the screams and came running from the other room. She smiled and gave Jason a kiss and a hug while he held Bailey. He looked into his wife's eyes and glimpsed the girl he had married. He recognized that living a loving life would make all the difference with his wife and family.

After dinner, Bailey and Becky joined Jason and Mike in the backyard to play soccer. After several minutes of play, Jason heard the baby crying from her walker on the patio and went to hold her. When he picked her up, he noticed the sun setting over the neighbor's house. He thought of his original vision as he looked back to the yard and saw Mike and Bailey laughing as Becky kicked the ball into the bushes. Hope filled his heart, and he felt better than he had in months. He wasn't used to acknowledging and paying attention to his feelings, but the training sessions with David were helping him to do this.

At their next session, David didn't follow up with Jason about homework. Jason's countenance showed that he was doing the homework steps and working the program. David started right into the evening's discussion.

"You have been addicted to viewing for a long time. When you first chose to live a loving life, you felt uncomfortable and probably still do to a lesser extent. This is typical when we change a habit or start something new. You felt stress, but it declined pretty rapidly as you continued. The feelings of discomfort will continue to diminish over the next two to three weeks. At that point, you'll feel close to normal and realize that your comfort zone has expanded to help you live a loving life.

"You'll still have temptations; in fact, I hope you created some thoughts that mimic temptations for your homework. Over time, you'll notice a decline in the number and intensity of the temptations you experience. There's no way around stress, but you can continue to feel stress and proceed anyway, recognizing that you are retraining yourself to achieve a wonderful vision.

"When you go through viewing and doing withdrawal, you can choose to be miserable, or you can choose to heal by embracing stress and temporary discomfort. In other words, acknowledge that the stress is a good thing. Choose the stress and choose the discomfort, recognizing that you are getting stronger and expanding your comfort zone.

"In the past, when you tried to quit viewing, you fought against the pain, stress, and discomfort of withdrawal. Now you'll be willing to embrace them because you know those feelings are leading to healing. The pain and discomfort are only temporary.

"Because this is so important, I want to discuss it further and emphasize it with an illustration. "You may not believe me when you look at my body now, but I used to train with weights in my younger days. I learned a very important principle. When I first started lifting weights, my muscles were so sore I could barely get out of bed the next day, and I had trouble walking for at least a week. But within a couple weeks, my muscles adapted and the soreness went away. If I had quit during the sore period, I never would have reached the new, expanded comfort zone of lifting.

"As I continued to train, I quickly learned that if I wanted to progress, I needed to push my muscles beyond their comfort zone and into painful territory. When I trained in this way—the pain wasn't too bad; I call it good pain—my muscles increased in strength and size much more rapidly than when I exercised pain-free.

"What do you think helped me power through the pain and discomfort?"

Jason quickly replied, "It must have been your vision."

David responded with a smile, "You're right. I had a vision of my appearance with ripped abs and defined muscles. So that you don't think it was all about vanity, I also had a vision of high energy and excellent athletic performance.

"I knew the pain, soreness, and overall discomfort would be temporary but essential for me to gain the strength and definition I desired and to perform athletically as I envisioned.

"So, the first concept of practice is, 'Expand your comfort zone, feel the pain, and know that you're growing.'" David wrote on the board as he spoke.

"Let's quickly move into practice concept number two, precision. A few years ago, I enjoyed a day skiing with a friend of mine. I noticed that he was a much better skier than I was, even though we had been at the same level a few years earlier. When I asked him how he improved so much while I stayed the same, he mentioned that he took lessons and worked on the suggestions from the instructor.

"The ski instructor watched him ski and then provided him with steps to improve his skiing. By following the specific steps in the precise way that the instructor directed, my friend's level of expertise rose quickly.

"You've received very specific steps from an experienced and, may I add, very good-looking instructor." David and Jason laughed, and David continued. "Now it's time to practice with precision." He wrote on the board, "Precision: Practice precisely to gain power on your way to mastery."

"When we practice specific instructions from an expert in the right way, we don't waste our practice but instead make it pay. Vince Lombardi, the legendary NFL coach, put it this way, 'Practice doesn't make perfect. Only perfect practice makes perfect.'

"I think it will be helpful to look at practicing things precisely, from both the how-to perspective and the how-not-to perspective. Let's first go over how not to practice. I think you'll see several ways that the how-nots lack precision. We'll label this 'Unhealthy Practice.'

"The first unhealthy practice is thinking that it's OK to cheat just once or thinking it's better to reduce viewing gradually. These are lies. Cheating just once doesn't just stop your progress cold; it causes you to start all over again and makes it much more difficult to achieve your goal. When you choose to cheat just once, you're choosing all the negative consequences of viewing, and you will need to start over. Let's go over some other components of unhealthy practice.

"Ignoring the temptation. If you try to ignore the temptation, it will fight and struggle for your attention. The temptation will linger and come back strongly to bite you. Acknowledging it makes it weaker.

"Treating the temptation as bad. There is no choice without temptation. It is OK to experience it and the emotion that accompanies it. After all, temptations are just thoughts. Everyone experiences them.

"Falling back into SAPS habits: Suppression, Avoidance, relying on Protection, and Substitution. These practices, common in unsuccessful programs, will lead to relapse. Whenever you begin to fall back into any of these habits, realize it's unhealthy and get back on track.

"Denying your ever-present freedom to choose. When you tell yourself that you must, you have to, you better, or you should, you're not telling the truth. You always have the freedom to choose.

"Focusing on the future or on the past. Thoughts of the future will bring anxiety. If you find yourself worrying about the future, tell yourself that your decision not to view pornography is for this instance only. You can choose differently next time. If you find yourself dredging up your viewer past, the familiar failure patterns and viewer self-image may come to mind. Always bring yourself back to the present and exercise your freedom to choose.

"Cheating on your vision statement. If you don't always state and feel your vision statement, it will become cloudy over time and lose its power. If your current vision statement starts to fade, it's time for you to reenergize it with emotion-charged language of a concrete, vivid vision that is directly related to your top five positive consequences.

"Skipping steps. When you practice, don't skip steps. When you get sloppy in your practice, you set yourself up for relapsing.

"Any questions about unhealthy practice?"

"No questions, but I think I have one to add. I'm not sure how to word it, but I noticed just prior to my relapse that I felt very confident. I thought that I had overcome the problem for good, that I didn't need to attend meetings any more. I think overconfidence and subsequent lack of practice led to my fall."

"Excellent. I think we can break this into two unhealthy practices. Let me try rephrasing them and see if we keep your meaning. In fact, I think the overconfidence component is so important that I'm going to expand it.

"Overconfidence leads to thinking that you no longer need to practice. It also typically precedes a relapse. When you become overconfident or you believe that you are cured, you are setting yourself up to skip steps (e.g., 'I don't need to go through the steps anymore—I'm cured') or to put yourself in SAPS mode. You also run the risk of rationalizing your way into overly tempting situations (e.g., 'Now that I'm cured, I can go to the strip club with colleagues but just stay in the back and not look').

"Failing to practice. Naturally, failing to practice is unhealthy and is often preceded by overconfidence. If you find yourself placing practice lower on your list of priorities, forgetting or stopping due to overconfidence, thinking you're too busy, or using other rationalizations, recognize it and recommit to practice.

"How did I do?"

"Great! You captured my meaning and added some other important aspects as well."

"As you know, I don't like to dwell on the negative, so let's quickly move on to the positive, 'Healthy Practice' steps:

"**Create a temptation in your mind.** Simply state, 'I want to view and do.' You may have to enter it in your calendar to remind yourself to do it. You'll then go through each of the AACV steps as if the temptation were real.

"**Acknowledge the created temptation immediately.** As we've discussed, deliberately acknowledging the temptation as it arrives is one of the keys to success. Don't let a temptation linger for even a moment, even if it comes from a thought that is self-created.

"**Quickly follow acknowledging with accepting.** If it seems redundant to accept your own created temptation, please do it anyway. Precise practice leads to a long-term loving life. Accept the temptation as normal—it happens to everyone—and move on to the next step.

"**Recognize and exercise your power to choose**. Just as you would with a real temptation, remember that your choice is for this instance only. Realizing that you can choose at any time to view and do will prevent feelings of deprivation that lead to relapse.

"**State and feel your vivid vision.** When you state your vision, feel it at the same time, even though you created the temptation. Emotions drive our decisions. The positive emotions evoked by your vision will power you past this and future temptations.

"So how do you like the practice session so far?"

Jason's response was immediate. "I've always known the value of practice, but this helps motivate me to do it right."

David looked surprised. "I'm glad you embraced practice so quickly. Many people struggle with the idea of creating a temptation or creating a thought that mimics a temptation. Viewers deal with temptation by succumbing to it so I can understand their reluctance to embrace creating one.

"Here's another sports analogy that helps reluctant "practicers" embrace creating temptations. Baseball players can only make so much progress by swinging the bat at baseballs pitched slowly. They can work on their mechanics but unless they practice batting balls pitched at game speed, they will not become good hitters.

The tremendous hand-eye coordination required to hit a baseball pitched at 95 miles per hour is not developed without practicing hitting baseballs pitched at 95 miles per hour. It is also not maintained without continuing to practice hitting 95-miles-per-hour pitches on a regular basis.

"Viewers can master the concepts of dealing with temptations but without continuing to practice at "game speed," they will be subject to relapse. Creating temptations is the equivalent of practicing hitting 95-mph-pitched baseballs.

"Now that you're doubly convinced of the need to create thoughts that mimic temptations for your practice to be effective, let me discuss another key aspect of precision. As you've shared your vision with me,

I've noticed slight changes in wording beyond the changes in meaning that we discussed.

Your vision is one of the most important parts of your recovery. It's important that you refine it so that the picture it paints in your mind is believable, vivid, and nearly tangible. Let's go over some tips to refine your vision.

"If the positive consequences upon which your vision is based are not grounded in truth, your mind will not believe you, and the vision will fail. If your vision is murky, grounded in abstract or hard-to-picture concepts, it loses its power. Use vivid words that evoke emotions and mind images.

"If your vision seems unreachable, it loses its power. This is the nearly tangible part of the vision. Craft your vision with positive consequences that are reachable in the short term. Fill it with words that make it feel real and close.

"Here's one other tip that can help empower your vision. If the vision rolls off your tongue easily and readily, you'll be more likely to use it as part of your AACV process. It doesn't need to be a poem, but if it sounds a little poetic, you will remember it, be proud of it, and recite it the same way each time. This allows it to become a part of you."

Jason agreed. "Powerful." I'll try to give my vision more ring and rhythm."

Note: *Please refer to* poweroverpornography.com/vision *for example vision statements. Please share your vision statement with the community while you view others.*

"Great. Let's move on." David wrote on the whiteboard again: "Repetition. Creating and maintaining a habit takes practice."

"Jason, I've found that some people don't believe that repetition helps. They don't see the value. When I come across this attitude, I can safely bet that the person showing it is going to have a much harder time succeeding.

"When lifting weights, if you don't repeat the exercises on a regular basis, you don't maintain muscle. If you don't repeat the AACV on a regular basis, you don't maintain your loving life. You become subject to relapsing and experiencing all its negative consequences.

"Now, let me repeat something that we covered in a prior session. I've tried to use the principle of repetition at various parts of our sessions as emphasis and to help you remember. After several days using this program, you discovered that the number of your temptations declined. This happens to everyone fully involved in the program. Because I emphasize the importance of practice, I encouraged you to create temptations out of thin air so that you can practice addressing them.

"During the first few weeks of the program, if you're not experiencing at least two to three temptations per day, then you should create temptations. As I recall, you were skeptical about creating thought temptations. Now that you've tried it, please tell me how you feel about it."

Jason thought for a moment. "It didn't make sense to me at first. I've always been told to avoid tempting situations and triggers. It seemed like I could get into trouble creating my own temptations."

David replied. "I understand how you felt. I used to think that way as well, and I spent many years thinking that the answer was avoidance and self-discipline. Now I realize that creating a fake temptation provides practice and helps cement choosing the best consequences.

"I spent too many years as a viewer and doer, so my reaction to triggers is wired in my brain. As I've explained before, in order to make a new reaction path in my brain, I needed and still need to practice. I've found that people unwilling to create their own temptation-mimicking thoughts often relapse after a few months. The old brain wiring takes over because they haven't practiced enough with the new reaction sequence."

"I understand," Jason responded. "I'm still adjusting to it, but I've created my own temptations as you suggested. I found that if I use the AACV card to address them immediately, I don't feel any more at risk of relapsing. I don't want to revert to my old viewing choices. I've learned that avoidance doesn't lead to healing and a life of love; it just puts off the inevitable relapse for a little while."

161

"That's a good way to phrase it. I'm going to remember that for helping future viewers. I'm glad you see it that way. In order to change the neural pathways of your brain and make the loving life your way of life, practice—including creating temptations and urges out of thin air—is essential. In fact, choosing to practice every day is like giving yourself an immunization against a deadly disease when you know you'll be among the infected.

"After three weeks, you can reduce the created temptations so that you are averaging one to two total temptations per day. You'll have enough practice under your belt by then that your job will be to maintain the pathways in your brain instead of building new ones.

"Do you recall when I told you that I'd been sober from pornography for twenty-two years?"

"Yeah. I was very impressed. I thought I was on that same path after my first foray into twelve-step programs, but I only lasted six months."

"One of the keys to my sobriety is practice. I still practice once per day dealing with temptations to view. Sometimes they're real, but most times I create temptations. I still occasionally have temptations come from unexpected sources, or triggers. Having practiced my daily AACV, I am able to deal with the new sources of urges just like the old ones.

"I'm afraid I would have relapsed had I not been practicing daily. If you're like everyone else who has been through this program, you'll require the same level of repetitive practice. This repetition will keep the vision from clouding over. It will further cement choosing the vision and positive consequences that you prefer. I hope you choose to practice every day so you can realize your vision and live a loving life."

Jason nodded his head in agreement, and David continued. "There are three specific daily practices that will keep the clouds away and keep you living a loving life."

David wrote, "Practice AACV twice per day, practice affirmations once per day, and practice relationship-building conversations and actions," on the board.

"We just went over how to practice AACV. We just covered affirmations and relationship-building actions recently so we won't plan to go over them again unless you have any questions."

Jason quickly responded, "I'm good."

David resumed. "Remember our initial discussion about clarity and how consequences of our actions become cloudy, so we have to clarify them to bring them to mind?"

Jason smiled. "Cloudy has become part of my vocabulary now when describing things I can't remember very well. I recall the discussion well. It was one of our early sessions, and I remember how new but powerful it felt to me."

"Well, over my twenty-two years of sobriety, I've adopted a specific way of practice that allows me to live a loving life. I've mentioned three of the critical steps to practice: attitude, precision, and repetition. Now I want to mention some of the others.

"I discovered early on that the hundred-day wall was real—"

"What is that?"

"We haven't discussed it directly yet, although we alluded to it when you brought up overconfidence and when we discussed the importance of practice. I, along with others who help individuals overcome pornography addiction, have found that once viewers achieve sobriety, a significant percentage relapse after ninety to a hundred days.

"We refer to this as the hundred-day wall. I'm not positive what causes it, but I suspect the core is overconfidence and subsequent lack of practice. Then a powerful, sudden, unexpected temptation hits. The person reverts back to the viewer brain wiring instead of following the AACV brain wiring, and relapses. Often, the initial relapse is followed by spiraling down in the shame cycle and multiple successive relapses, leading directly to a life full of misery and all the negative consequences we've discussed.

"I sometimes refer to the wall as the hundred-day wall of clouds. I like to think that the daily practice keeps some of the clouds away, but the full program becomes cloudy over time, and the potential for relapse sneaks in.

"There are five steps we've instituted as part of practice that break down the hundred-day wall of clouds and build toward mastery and the all-important maintenance of mastery, or keeping the clouds away. Just like a professional athlete has to keep practicing to keep his skills sharp, so do we. Mastering them once and then forgetting to practice them would result in their atrophy, similar to how a quarterback's ability to throw to receivers would atrophy without practice."

David wrote these steps on the board as he stated them. "First, be aware of the hundred-day wall. Once you know about it, you can bolster your practice when you start drifting or becoming overconfident. Second, institute scenario practice; third, institute program review to remove cloudiness; fourth, become involved in the community; and fifth, read related stories, updates, new research, and practice tips on a monthly basis. This will provide additional help and motivation to stay on the path of living a loving life."

Jason said, "I was feeling pretty comfortable about the first three practice steps, but now it seems pretty complicated. Plus, I'm a little worried about this hundred-day wall coming up."

"Remember that the choice is always yours, and you can choose to view anytime you want. You're not at the hundred-day point, so you don't need to worry about it now. Bring yourself back to the present and concern yourself with this moment and your choices.

"Also, remember that forewarned is forearmed. You now know a failure path that many have trod before. If they would have known about this path, they may have avoided it. You now have the practice steps of the success path. I fully anticipate that by using these practice steps day-by-day, you'll choose your vision and won't even notice the wall. It will be more like a hundred-day speed bump for you."

Jason seemed reassured, so David continued. "Let's address the complicated nature of the practice. I think once you understand the practice steps, you'll see how they can flow naturally and don't take much more than a few minutes per day. It's mostly practicing concepts and exercises that you've learned in the program already.

"Take number two, 'institute scenario practice.' This means you create temptation-mimicking thoughts involving different scenarios that you can imagine happening at some point. Here are some example scenarios to consider: A friend invites you to go to an R-rated movie that has nudity; an e-mail you receive has a nude (or almost nude) photo and a link to an associated website; you notice a pretty, scantily clad woman at the store; you receive free access to HBO or another premium movie service at home; you travel to Las Vegas for a business convention and have access to pornographic movies, strip clubs, and so forth.

"These scenarios could be triggers for you, but you will want to think of your own temptation scenarios. Each viewer has similar triggers but also tends to have ones that are particularly tempting to him or her. If you experience or imagine a scenario that is particularly tempting to you, including fantasies, you should include that in your scenarios.

"Once you've listed your scenarios, go through two of them as AACV practice once every other week. By practicing the scenario temptations, you will be prepared for unexpected, strong temptations.

> Note: *Scenario practice is such an important component that it has its own webpage. Please refer to* poweroverpornography.com/scenarios *to review and select scenarios. Please share some of your suggested scenarios to help others.*

"Remembering to practice scenarios once every two weeks can be difficult, so I suggest you schedule the practice sessions on your calendar for the entire next year. Scenario practice should take only five minutes or less, once every other week. A simple calendar reminder can prompt you to do it. Does this seem doable?"

"Now that you've explained it, it seems doable. I can see how this type of practice will prepare me to face a variety of temptations."

"Great. Let's move on to the next one, program review.

"The major parts of the program include clarifying consequences, acknowledging and accepting temptations, exercising the power to choose, developing and choosing a vivid vision, stating affirmations, working on relationships, and practicing. We've discovered that cloudiness returns to consequences when there is no practice. Cloudiness also returns to many other aspects of the program if regular reviews are not performed.

"I hope you've noticed that the homework includes review of prior exercises. This is to make sure that the critical parts of the program remain in your conscious mind so that you can use them to take power back from viewing pornography.

"By regularly reviewing key parts of the program, you'll remain strong on your path to living a loving life. In this case, regular means a once-per-month repeat of a session of your choice so that you are reviewing the entire program over a one-year period. In essence, it's thirty to sixty minutes per month, regularly scheduled on your calendar. How does that sound?"

Jason responded slowly, "It seems doable, but it also seems like this practice is getting rather extensive. I can see the merit in reviewing, but it seems so fresh in my mind that the monthly review time seems like overkill."

David smiled as he said, "You do a great job of knowing your heart and providing honest feedback. This allows me to customize our sessions and make them more impactful for you.

"Let me address your concern. You've spent years as a viewer and doer. The residual habit remains until your response is so practiced that it happens automatically. Once the things you've learned in POP become automatic, they won't stay that way without practice.

The details and reasons are prominent in your mind right now, but they will fade over time, and you will become more susceptible to relapse. The recommendations for practice are based on the experiences of other viewers, both successful and not. I hope you'll trust this basis and experience the long-term success you want.

"If I ever sound a little heavy-handed and your inner rebel begins to come out, recognize that it's always your choice to practice. An alternative to the once per month session of your choice is an annual review of the entire program. Please choose the option that works best for you."

Jason nodded and David continued, "Becoming involved in the community is a success factor that we borrowed directly from twelve-step programs, such as Alcoholics Anonymous. The support you find from other people experiencing the same addiction has healing power. You'll take heart that you're not alone and that others are healing from viewing. You'll receive power from knowing that others are successfully working the program and living a loving life.

"I know that many of our ex-viewers have a difficult time getting together in person, so I've set up blogs and online forums to gather a community. I'm new at online stuff, but so far it seems to be helping. I invite you to contribute to as well as learn from others in the POP community.

"Another way to gain power from community is to attend twelve-step programs."

Note: *We make practice easy for you. Please sign up for our practice program at* poweroverpornography.com/practice. *You will receive regular e-mails with specific practice steps and suggestions to help you maintain your loving life. Also, don't forget to join the community by exploring the forums at* poweroverpornography.com/forums.

"The last practice tip for making the hundred-day wall into a hundred-day speed bump is less concrete, but it's important. Although we've characterized it as 'Read monthly stories, updates, research, and practices that boost motivation,' we can summarize it as, 'Stay in the healing zone of the program to stay motivated.'

"Once you register on the website, the community and I will stay in touch with you and send you additional information and research, such as stories of others, new research findings, and program changes. These communications will help you improve your existing practice as we discover other success paths.

Jason responded, "I like self-development programs. I know this is different, but my experience with those programs helps me see the value of the regular motivational communication.

"When I've been involved in self-improvement programs before, I've started strong and then lost interest over time and gradually stopped. I can really see the merit of staying connected with new research and stories to keep motivated and to stay on track."

"Great. We're going to end our discussion now so you can go home and enjoy the evening with your family. We've covered a lot of aspects of practice today, and you'll need some time to absorb them and set up your plans. Next time, we'll discuss traveling and other special situations and how to deal with them.

"Remember, mastery requires practice, and practice helps you live a loving life."

Homework for Practice, the Power over Relapse:

1. Write the following statement and say it out loud (in your mind if you're not in a private place).
   a. When I feel discomfort, stress, or anxiety, I embrace the feeling, realizing I'm growing stronger and my comfort zone is expanding.
2. Write out two to five scenarios that would present temptations. Schedule five minutes every other week to run through AACV practice for two of those scenarios.
3. Schedule thirty to forty-five minutes per month for the next year to review a session of the program. Alternatively, schedule a complete program review once per year. Choose to honor the schedule.
4. Sign up for the online community and participate.
5. Read stories, research, and new practice methods to stay motivated.

Whiteboard Chapter 15

Practice:

- Attitude: Expand your comfort zone, feel the pain, and know that you're growing.
- Precision: Practice precisely to gain power on your way to mastery.
- Repetition: Creating and maintaining a habit takes practice.
  - Practice AACV twice per day.
  - Practice affirmations once per day.
  - Practice relationship-building conversations and actions.

Hundred-Day Wall: Power over Relapse

- Be aware that the hundred-day wall is coming.
- Institute scenario practice.
- Institute regular program review to keep clouds away.
- Become involved in the community.
- Read monthly stories, updates, research, and practices that boost motivation.

CHAPTER 16:

Travel and Special Situations

Jason was excited to get home. Tonight was Mike's first soccer game of the season. Since starting POP, Jason felt more like a real father.

Mike was waiting on the front stoop as Jason drove in the driveway. "Dad, let's go to the game. I don't want to be late!" Mike shouted as he ran to the car.

"Hello to you too, buddy. The game doesn't start for two hours. We'll make sure we're on time, but I want to change first and eat a little."

"Well, hurry up."

"All right. I think our team is ready, and I'm excited to see how you do in your first game. Let's go eat dinner."

When the referee blew the whistle signaling the end of regulation, the score was tied three to three. Each team then exchanged penalty kicks. Mike's team made three of five kicks. The other team made four.

Mike was one of the two players on his team who missed their penalty kicks, and cried as he came off the field. Jason quickly put his arm around him but didn't say anything. It seemed like the right thing to do.

After Mike started to calm down, he whimpered. "I lost the game for my team."

"I think you're one of the reasons the team even made it to penalty kicks. You played a good game, but I understand how it hurts. It's OK to feel sad about it.

"Once we get home, I'll remind you of all the great passes and shots you made, and you'll feel a lot better." Mike didn't say anything as they walked to the car. As she loaded Bailey and Nicole into the car, Becky told Mike that he played a good game.

Despite the loss and Mike's sadness, Jason was excited about the game and proud that he had not yelled at the refs. *That may be a first for me*, he thought. *Living a loving life seems to be working in other areas of my life besides my family relationships.*

At their next meeting, David greeted Jason. "Welcome to your last regular session. How are you feeling about the program, your progress, and your outlook?"

"Interesting you should ask, but I'm not sure what you mean by 'regular.'"

"I'm sure you did your homework, but let's review it. Last time we discussed practice and life beyond the scheduled program sessions. There are a number of ongoing practices—pun intended—that will keep you living a loving life. Why don't you share your homework experience with me?"

"Oh, I understand what you're referring to. Yes, I did the homework, and I realize how important ongoing practice is to success.

"I'm still experiencing one or more temptations per day, so I'm creating more, at least two per day. It's working. I run through the AACV process and feel more power each time, but don't worry. I'm not getting cocky."

"Good. Tell me about your other practice experience."

"Well, the affirmations, which at first seemed hokey, are working. I smile each morning after I say them, and I am feeling better. I say them to myself in the mirror while I'm shaving. Unless I grow a beard, I'll remember to say them each day. I walk out of the bathroom each morning with increased confidence. I've become a fan of affirmations.

"The relationship practice went a little more slowly. I haven't had any serious relationship discussions with Becky, but I'm listening better and trying to talk about more serious subjects. I think I can help rebuild the relationship over time. It is kind of scary though. I've never been good at engaging in deep conversations."

"You'll get better with practice, and your relationship with Becky can and should evolve into a source of great joy and happiness for both of you. What about the scenario practices?"

"I felt a little funny at first, trying to imagine myself in potentially compromising situations, but I feel like it helps me be prepared for temptations that wouldn't occur every day. I have my review sessions scheduled for the whole year, and I am looking forward to engaging in the online community and hearing more from you on a regular basis.

"You mentioned last time that the scenario practice can help me when I'm confronted with a temptation that is different and possibly stronger from what I encounter normally. I'm not overly worried about it, but I am interested in learning from others in the POP community about the temptations they face. If they ring true to me as possible temptations, then I can include them in my scenario practice.

"I think if I would have known how to practice and then done it every day after my initial success with the twelve-step program, I wouldn't have relapsed. I can see how practice is vital to living a loving life. Thank you for teaching it to me and for committing to help me as I go forward."

"It's been my pleasure. As the saying goes, the teacher always learns more than the student. These sessions have been great for me to practice and relearn the POP concepts and exercises. Anything else?"

"This isn't practice-related, but remember when I told you about my experience with the leader of my church?"

"Yes. As I recall, your last interaction wasn't that great."

"Right. Well, I spoke with him again on Sunday. I felt, based upon my beliefs, that I needed to confess my relapse to him. I dreaded it, but it felt like the kind of uncomfortable feeling that I could feel and do it anyway. I did it, and it was a good experience. As I knelt beside my bed that night in prayer, I felt a great sense of happiness come over me, and I realized that my happiness in general has increased.

"I feel like I'm forgiven of my viewing and doing. In the past, my attempts at confession and repentance to God were halfhearted because I felt like I was going to relapse in the future. It wasn't sincere, even though I wanted more than anything to stop. This time was different. I felt sincere. I believed that now I can choose to stay porn-free and live a loving life. It was a remarkable spiritual experience.

"Many years ago, I heard a new convert speak of his experience in embracing God. He described how he thought he was happy and that his life was just fine before his conversion. He then said that since he found God, he experienced a new, higher plane of happiness that he didn't know existed.

"That description stayed with me and came to mind again after my prayer experience on Sunday. I realized that my happiness quotient has increased since I've been learning from you and practicing my AACV, affirmations, and other parts of the program. My love for my family, especially my wife, is stronger and deeper. My critical nature has transformed so that I am more accepting and less easily provoked to anger. I feel the Spirit of God in my life in a way that I haven't felt in years or maybe ever.

"That's the long answer to how I'm doing. The short answer is that I'm doing great."

"I'm glad you shared your experience with me, Jason. We briefly discussed the deep shame and tremendous hits to self-esteem that are natural consequences of viewing. We didn't discuss the big hits to your relationship with God, but that is also a natural consequence.

"This program works for those who have faith in God and for those who don't. I believe in God and actively practice my religion, but I respect those with different beliefs. I just want to help everyone realize the positive consequences of living a loving life.

"Now that you've shared a bit of your religious beliefs with me, I'll share some of mine with you. I believe that all of us are God's children, and I believe He is offended that any of his children would be used by pornographers. I believe that when we view pornography and masturbate, we are misusing one of the greatest powers he's given us as his children, that of creating life. I think His Spirit withdraws from us when we engage in viewing and doing.

"When you feel that you are violating God's commandments, you naturally pull away from Him. He is always there and willing to help, but you feel—rightly so—that you are not in good standing with him, so you have a harder time connecting with Him and His Spirit.

"The idea I mentioned a moment ago, that misusing the gift and power of creation causes God's Spirit to withdraw from us, is a powerful thought that I experience when you and others discuss the consequences of viewing and doing.

"Almost all men and women discover that the loss of love in their hearts is a natural consequence. I believe this loss is partly due to having less access to the Spirit of God because of misuse of the power to create life.

"The deep shame and low self-esteem make it difficult for you to love others and to maintain strong, loving relationships with anyone, even those closest to you. They also make it difficult for you to maintain a strong relationship with God and to feel his direction in your life."

Jason nodded, feeling the power of David's words.

"I don't generally discuss my beliefs throughout this program even though they are strongly held. My desire is to help everyone, and I worry that those who believe otherwise may reject the message if they disagree with the messenger.

"On the other hand, I would be ungrateful if I didn't acknowledge God's hand in this program and mention that the principles upon which it is based will work. I give all the credit and glory to God. If you're interested, we can meet again, and I can lay out the principles from a spiritual perspective."

Note: *Please refer to* poweroverpornography.com/spiritualprinciples *to read some of the specific spiritual principles that apply to the POP system.*

"I would like that."

"I'm glad to see that your progress toward living a loving life is paying dividends for you already. You'll certainly have bumps in the road in your relationships along the way because you're human, but living a loving life instead of being a viewer will make those bumps feel smaller.

"Now, let's talk about travel and special situations this week."

David wrote, "The challenges of travel."

"First of all, Jason, do you travel much?"

"I'm mostly local, but I have spent several days at a time at clients' locations in different states. I usually travel two or three times per year to training seminars."

"In the past, how was your viewing habit when you traveled?"

"A lot worse than when I'm not traveling."

"I suspected it might be. Let's explore why and address what to do about it."

David turned to the whiteboard and wrote, "High stress."

"Do you generally experience greater stress when you're traveling?"

"I suppose so. The wait for security, worrying about late planes, dealing with crowds and unfamiliar places, and having so much of the travel experience out of my control add to the stress."

"What was one of the number-one ways you chose to relieve stress in the past?"

"Viewing and doing."

"Now you know that viewing and doing actually create more stress and put you in the cycle of increased stress and increased shame that made your life and relationships miserable.

"When the added stress of travel hits you, before you know it you can succumb to viewing and doing. The key is preparing for it so you'll recognize it and be able to exercise your AACV process.

"Before we get into applying the AACV process, let's make sure you're prepared for the other issues you face with travel."

David wrote, "Different environment."

"You're used to practicing the AACV process in your home and work environment, and you are seeing results with your most important relationships and probably with your work performance. When you're faced with a different environment, the temptation can creep up on you without your recognizing it. When this happens, you may not respond immediately with the acknowledge-and-accept process.

"One of the main reasons for imagining tempting scenarios is to prepare you for different environments. I hope that business travel remains one of those scenarios for you. As long as you realize you'll be in a different environment and that the temptation may take different forms because of that, you'll be able to recognize, acknowledge, and accept it. In essence, in a different environment, you need to add the R for recognize to the beginning of the process: RAACV."

David wrote on the whiteboard: "Low chance of getting caught."

"When you're alone in your hotel room with adult movies available on TV and no possibility of being discovered on your usual adult websites, the temptations may take on an added strength. These conditions could be accompanied by the lies that say, 'Just this once won't hurt,' 'I'm not hurting anyone but myself,' or even 'No one will know.'

"By the way, I'm not a fan of labeling pornography 'adult.' There is nothing about viewing pornography that is adult. The adult path is the nonaddictive path, not the artificial, relationship-destroying path. The mark of adult behavior is the delay of immediate gratification in exchange for greater joy in the future. Childish behavior is satisfying current urges regardless of future consequences.

"You already know that 'just this once' is a lie, maybe the biggest one. I think you realize that choosing to view just once will put you back in the downward spiral. You always have the right to choose at every instance so that you won't feel denied or deprived, but if you hear in your head, "Just this once won't hurt," tell yourself the truth—that it will hurt—and then put yourself into AACV mode so you can choose your vision."

As he talked, David wrote: "Pie on the windowsill—strong temptation close at hand."

"Back in the olden days," David said, smiling, "One of the common illustrations for a warning against tempting others was the story of a mother who put her pie on the windowsill to cool after taking it out of the oven. When the children helped themselves to the pie after the mother instructed them to not touch it, the blame shifted to the mother for introducing such a strong temptation that the children could not resist.

"As you can guess, I don't like the analogy. The children give their power to the mother when they say the temptation was too strong. If they were prepared for it, they could have dealt with it.

"The closeness of the temptation when traveling is related to this. It's right in front of you in a way that you are not used to confronting on a daily basis. Once you recognize this difference and realize that it may come quickly and strongly, you'll be prepared for it.

"Now that you know some of the differences in temptations while traveling, you'll be prepared to deal with them. Not only will you be able to add 'recognize' to the AACV formula but you will want to add some vividness to your vision. When you suspect the temptation will come in different forms and more strongly, you'll want to focus on overwhelming it with a powerful vision.

"I've developed the travel formula specifically for those who travel frequently or who may find themselves in high-stress situations. It has been refined as a result of seeing what works for frequent travelers.

"On the day you travel, make time for the following steps. Plan to do them before you arrive at your destination. Some viewer and doer travelers prefer to do it on the plane, while others take a few minutes in the morning before they walk out the door. Consider this formula your 'away-game' practice.

"First, write down your top five negative consequences. Read them to yourself at least three times each.

"Next, write down your top five positive consequences. Read them to yourself at least three times each.

"Although you've written both the negative and positive consequences before, write them again as part of the formula. Writing uses more of your senses, takes greater action, and helps cement the consequences in your brain. Reading them to yourself multiple times will help them stay near the front of your mind instead of the back of your mind (they become less cloudy). Remember how important repetition is.

"Rewrite your vision. Because you've practiced reciting it multiple times—remember the power of repetition—this will be easy for you to do. Use this rewriting as a time to vividly picture it in your mind. If it's losing some of its vividness, tweak it to bring it back to life.

"After that, close your eyes and rehearse the mental picture of your vision three times. The vision will grow in strength, and the visualization exercise will leave you happy, relaxed, and confident.

"Recite your affirmations three times. They will increase your confidence and your self-esteem. The affirmations keep you in the mind-set of who you really are instead of who you used to be.

"For your homework, please write the away-game practice steps on a note card and put it in a pocket of your travel bag. This will help remind you of the steps to take to prepare for traveling."

Jason smiled. "The rule of five. These steps make good sense to me for business trips."

David smiled back and said, "There are other special situations beyond traveling that can put you in situations with viewing or doing temptations that you haven't experienced before. The best way to manage them is to create scenarios for them and walk through the AACV process with each one. In essence, when you undertake your regular scenario practice, spend the first couple minutes creating one or two new scenarios that you can imagine yourself experiencing.

"As you suggested earlier, you'll learn of other scenarios when you join our online community and see what others have experienced. Now that you've completed a scenario exercise, are there other scenarios you can imagine yourself experiencing?"

"Here are a few situations that I thought of. Becky received a call from her mother this week saying that her dad will be in the hospital for surgery in a couple weeks. She thinks her mother was hinting that it would be nice for Becky to come for a few days or even a full two weeks.

"I am concerned about how her being gone will affect my viewing and doing. In the past, viewing picked up—sometimes pretty ferociously—if Becky was out of town."

"Go on."

"I may start feeling deprived and feel like I deserve to satisfy my sexual desires by viewing and doing. I think if I go through the scenario of her being gone and focusing on my freedom to choose, I can handle this one."

"Great scenario, and good job catching the way it will try to lie to you about your freedom to choose. Any others that come to mind?"

"In the past, I would fantasize about a girlfriend from college. I was initially surprised that I haven't experienced that one recently, but I think my increased love for my wife has helped. I'm not naïve enough to think it's gone for good.

"I think instead of acknowledging a desire to view and do, I'll acknowledge and accept a temptation to have sex with her. It seems a little crass, but that is how the temptation hits, and I think I need to acknowledge it correctly."

"It almost seems like you're teaching me now. I think your scenarios are excellent, and acknowledging the actual temptation is an important step in killing it. You seem to understand quite well how to handle special situations or temptations with scenario practice. This is important as you imagine new types of temptation scenarios in your weekly practice sessions.

"Let's talk a little more about fantasy. You just described one that periodically hits you regarding an old girlfriend. Most viewers have a difficult time not recalling images of past views or other fantasies, some similar to what you described.

"When trying to stop viewing, many viewers resort to fantasizing with past images in their minds. Other viewers will fantasize with celebrities or others they may know.

"Viewers often see fantasies as the smoking alternative to alcohol for alcoholics, like we talked about in a previous session.

"Many viewers rationalize that trading actual viewing or doing for fantasizing means they are not in their addiction. What do you think?"

Jason thought for a moment. "It seems like fantasies are just a form of substitution. The temptation hasn't been dealt with directly with AACV. In the past, when I began to fantasize because I thought it was a better alternative to viewing and doing, I felt like I had started on the path, or cycle, and viewing and doing was inevitable.

"Are the consequences of fantasizing the same as actually viewing and doing?"

David didn't answer the question but instead asked, "What do you think? Did you suffer from the same consequences when you fantasized?"

Jason answered quickly. "Yeah. I think I was letting my viewing mind try to rationalize that fantasizing was different and not as bad. But now that I recall my own experiences, I think the consequences are probably the same—maybe not as severe, but still the same."

"Based upon my work with many other viewers, I think you're right. When a viewer starts fantasizing, he or she is on the road to viewing and begins to suffer the same consequences. What should be done when fantasies of past viewing, other pretty girls, celebrities, past girlfriends, or of any other sexual situation pop into your mind?"

"That's simple. I should practice AACV, just like with temptations to view and do."

"Right. Fantasy is just another type of temptation and should be dealt with the same way."

"I just have one other item to cover before we review the whole program. Generally, when we learn something that changes our lives, we like to share it with other people. As you know, helping others overcome their addiction is one of the steps of twelve-step programs. However, because of the potential embarrassment that results for people when they admit they are a viewer, we tend to see less sharing of the POP principles.

"I see the lives of many people destroyed because of pornography. I've tried fighting it at the source but to no avail. I believe the spread of pornography will only get more aggressive, and avoiding it will become more and more difficult. So, my focus now is to get the message of this program into as many hands as I can so that lives and relationships can be restored and so that love and confidence can replace misery and low self-image.

"Can you think of any ways you can share this program with others? I know you have a full-time job and are busy with family and church responsibilities, so I'm not asking you to become a full-time teacher. But helping others is an important step for you to keep living a loving life."

Jason thought for a moment and then said, "I can think of a few ways to share it. I am one of those people who are deeply embarrassed by their viewing, so I don't want to share my story in public. But I can see a few ways to share it in other ways. I feel strongly that this has changed my life. I was headed for a divorce or a life of misery and the potential loss of my job. Now I have hope again. And I want to share it with others who may be suffering like I was.

"Here are some of my thoughts on ways I can share. I can mention it to my church leaders so they can explore the program with you and refer viewers and doers. I know many of my leaders in the past had little clue how to help.

"When I hear men joke around about looking at porn, I know they realize deep down that it's wrong and is hurting them. I could mention that porn is a serious problem and that I've heard of many people quitting porn through this program.

"I can post an anonymous flyer on the bulletin boards at work and at church in the hopes that someone may notice it and call you for help.

"I plan to get involved on the community pages of your website and other similar websites to share my experiences and future learning so that others can learn as well. I'll probably do it anonymously though.

"I'm sure I'll think of other ways to share as well."

David responded by saying, "One benefit that comes from sharing and looking for opportunities to share is the top-of-mind experience you have. Do you remember how becoming a sponsor and helping others is a key step in the twelve-step programs? Well, it's one of those fundamental truths that when you help another, you are helped. So I encourage you to share the program with others and find new and different ways to share it. You will benefit just as much, if not more, than they will.

"You didn't find me by coincidence. I was where you were, and someone else helped me. By helping you, I keep myself humble and assist my own ongoing recovery. I hope you take the opportunity to do the same."

David stuck out his hand, and Jason grabbed it. "Congratulations, Jason. You completed the program. As you've followed the steps, raised questions, and completed the homework, I've noticed the changes in you. You have the swagger back in your step, so to speak.

"When I saw you after your relapse, you seemed lost and not very confident. Now you seem like you're not only living a loving life but loving the life you're living. You're realizing some of the positive consequences you identified early in the program.

"This is the greatest payoff to me, to see you make such positive changes after you had almost given up. To see the light come back into your eyes and to see the hope return is very gratifying. Thanks for sticking with the program, even when parts of it seemed counterintuitive."

Jason stood and hugged David quickly and said, "Thank you." He was afraid that if he said any more, he would cry. He felt like he was truly living a loving life.

David handed Jason a few pages and said, "Here is the summary of the program. Please read it as your last homework assignment (Please see Chapter 18 for the summary). I'll keep in touch and expect you to as well. Have fun with your family tonight."

Whiteboard Chapter 16

The Challenges of Travel:
- High stress
- Different environment
- Low chance of getting caught
- Pie on the windowsill—strong temptation close at hand

CHAPTER 17:

What about Relapse?

"Hi, Jason, it's good to hear from you. I'm glad you decided to call me. I've been thinking about you and your progress with the POP program. How's it going?"

"Hi, David, it's good to hear your voice. You sacrificed a lot to help me understand and implement the program. I feel like a new man."

After an awkward pause, David asked, "But…?"

"Oh, I'm sorry, David. I haven't relapsed or anything, but I can't get one concern out of my mind, so I thought I would call and ask your advice. Is now a good time?"

"I consider you a friend, Jason, so I'm glad you called. I'm honored that you want to share your concern with me, and I'll do whatever I can to help. It's a great time for me to talk. What's been bothering you?"

"I've been experiencing some fear the last few days about future relapsing. I know it probably sounds strange, but I have this nagging concern in my mind. If I can live a life of love for six months and then relapse while working a twelve-step program, what makes me think I won't do the same with the POP program? I haven't been able to shake this concern."

"My guess is that you probably know the answer, but sometimes we all need to talk a question through with someone to coax the answer out of our minds and give it some clarity. You just finished a program that provided some great learning, but it also contained a lot of new information that is hard to absorb all at once.

"Let me ask a few questions first, and then we'll proceed. What do you feel are the main differences between how your loving life is going now versus how it went before?"

"I feel a little more relaxed now, especially with the power to choose differently if I want to in the future."

"Do you really feel you have the power to choose to view and do whenever you want—that your choice to live a loving life is for this instance only?"

"I thought I did, but now that you phrase it like that, maybe I wasn't feeling it. Maybe I felt like my choice was forever. I can see how that would contribute to my fears of future relapse."

"What about your practice? Have you kept up with your schedule?"

"I'm good at the daily practice, but I missed the last restating of consequences. I thought that the consequences were still pretty fresh in my mind, so I should be able to skip one time. I am keeping up with AACV practice though."

"I'm glad to hear you're keeping up with the AACV practice. I hope you're also getting a sense for why I'm asking these specific questions. The POP program is usually relapse-free when executed correctly.

"Because of the way our minds work, practice is an essential part of the program. Our minds are created in a way that long-term consequences and visions are both in a constant state of fading. In order to keep the consequences clear of clouds and to keep our visions tangible and in the front of our minds, we need to regularly rehearse and review them.

"Life wouldn't be much of a challenge if we were always able to weigh all the consequences at their full weights before making decisions. As it is, we give more weight to the consequences with short-term gratification because the longer term consequences become cloudy and receive less and less weight with time.

"By regularly reviewing the consequences, we keep the clouds away. They stay clear and vivid in the forefront of our minds so that we can make a logical, sound choice that is in line with our long-term best interests.

"The two most common failure paths are letting the clouds come back and overconfidence, both of which are thwarted with active practice." David asked Jason to imagine the statements being written on the whiteboard.

Jason chuckled. He was already picturing this.

"We let the clouds in when we fail to review and rehearse the negative and positive consequences list or fail to keep the vision fresh, vivid, and tangible."

"In fact, reviewing and rehearsing form just part of the keys to staying with the loving life. The other factor is recognizing that choosing is more complicated than just choosing an action. We've seen some relapses occur because people shift from choosing consequences to choosing actions. Remember, your chances of success go way up when you choose consequences.

"Some recovering viewers can believe that they are healed and no longer have to use the AACV process. When they stop practicing AACV, they often encounter a temptation that happens in a different place or a different way than normal or that comes more strongly than usual. The overconfidence that led to them abandoning the AACV process with every temptation proves to be their downfall, and they relapse.

Please keep in mind that all of us are vulnerable to temptation and to falling. When we remember that we're vulnerable, we remember to practice. The most common consequence of overconfidence is failure to practice. When we feel like we're healed, we don't think we need to continue practicing.

"As you know, AACV is the essence of the program and the backbone of living a loving life. But practice is just as essential to living a loving life. When people religiously follow the POP practice schedule they avoid relapse.

"Did you put all the practice sessions on your calendar?"

"The practice sessions were kind of complicated with daily, weekly, and monthly times, so I may have missed some. I can see now that they are vital and will go a long way to helping me rid myself of the concern over future relapse. I'll get them scheduled."

"Great. How do you feel now?"

"I feel much better. My freedom to choose is reenergized, and I'll practice tonight to push the clouds away."

"Here's one other thing to keep in mind: relapse is not part of the program. If you do relapse, stop your spiral as soon as you can by starting the program from the beginning. Don't skip the homework. The writing exercises, especially of the consequences and vision, really help."

Whiteboard Chapter 17

Failure Paths
- Letting the clouds in
  - Not reviewing consequences
  - Not keeping vision fresh and vivid
- Overconfidence
  - Believing that you're no longer vulnerable
  - Not practicing

Note: *We've discovered that the most effective method of overcoming pornography addiction is the completion of our intensive seminars, followed by our online course combined with the e-mail practice program. Preliminary results indicate a 90% success rate or higher. Second best is the online course combined with practice program. Third best is the practice program alone. Success rates drop when the practice program is excluded and drop further when the online course is not completed. We encourage you to attend a live intensive seminar if you can. If you are unable or unsure about doing that at this time, enroll and complete the online course and subscribe to the practice program in order to ensure your success at living a loving life. You may find the course at* poweroverpornography.com/course. *You may find the Practice Program Subscription page at* poweroverpornography.com/practice

CHAPTER 18:

Summary of the Program Steps

Step 1: Commit to finishing the program. When you commit yourself in faith, admitting that you can't do it yourself, you unlock the power of commitment to help you overcome viewing.

Step 2: Clarify the negative consequences. Determine the truthful consequences of viewing pornography. Use reliable sources and stories. Narrow the list to the top five consequences that you most want out of your life. By deliberately clarifying the consequences before taking action, we increase our chances of choosing wisely.

Step 3: Clarify the positive consequences of living a loving life. Narrow this list to the top five positive consequences you most want in your life. When you review your consequences, you'll benefit much more from the positive ones. The more clear, positive, and emotion-filled they are, the better. Remember, you can choose your actions, but you can't choose different consequences than the actions dictate.

Step 4: Create your vision using your positive consequences list. Remember the James Allen quotation: "He who cherishes a beautiful vision, a lofty ideal in his heart, will one day realize it." Your vision will provide tremendous power. For your mind to see your vision clearly, it needs to be well-defined, vivid, and positive. Make it focused on the benefits to you, not others. Keep it simple (KIS).

Step 5: Acknowledge all temptations. Remember Victor Frankl's words, "Between stimulus and response there is a space. In that space is our power to choose our response. In our response lies our growth and our freedom." Immediately acknowledge every temptation plainly, directly, and specifically.

Step 6: Accept all temptations as normal. Temptations come to all; they are not bad, and they should not cause guilt.

Step 7: Recognize and exercise your power to choose. Choices are for a single instance only. You are free to choose differently in every instance. This concept is a key to the program and a key to your power. Choosing vision, positive consequences, benefits, and results gives you power. When you tell yourself that you must, have to, better, ought to, should, or are supposed to, you are denying your freedom to choose and thus lose your power.

Step 8: Use the AACV process to confront and deal with every viewing and doing temptation and any related ones. Write it down and recite it with every temptation without exception.

1. *Acknowledge* the temptation in first person ("I want to view and do…").
2. *Accept* the temptation as normal ("…and it's OK").
3. Exercise your freedom to *choose* ("I am free to choose, and I choose…").
4. Choose your customized, positive *vision*.

Step 9: Embrace the stress, anxiety and discomfort (SAD) of change. Overcoming long-held habits like viewing and doing involves some stress, anxiety and discomfort. Recognize that these feelings are natural and part of starting to live a loving life. Like the title of the self-help book, "feel the fear and do it anyway."

Step 10: Recognize and reject the power takers or failure paths: SAPS and doing it for others.

Suppress: When you attempt to suppress the temptation with your own willpower, it will increase in power and refuse to leave.

Avoid: When you attempt to avoid triggers and temptations instead of confronting them directly with the AACV process, the temptation does not go away but increases in power.

Protect: When you rely upon protection, such as computer filters, disconnecting the Internet, and so forth, you have not confronted and dealt with the temptation, so it will not go away. However, please use protection for other people who may access your electronics.

Substitute: When you try to substitute another thought or action for the temptation, the temptation gains power and comes back strongly because it has not been confronted and dealt with.

Do the program for yourself, not for others. Others will benefit, but the power comes from doing it for you.

Step 11: Recognize the lie in rationalizations. When you provide reasons for your viewing and doing, they are generally not true and not worth it. It's important to recognize them as lies. Refer to the chapter "Why Do We View Pornography?" for detailed examples.

Step 12: Repair the damage. Use affirmations on a daily basis to rapidly repair the damage viewing and doing did to your self-image. Set and achieve worthy goals to get back on track to living a loving life.

Step 13: Repair the relationship. True intimacy is an important part of your relationship with your spouse, and it is formed over years of trust, respect, kindness, and affection. Those not married can work on the foundations of true intimacy to improve their future relationship. Practice listening, sharing, being dependable, being honest, and demonstrating your love.

Step 14: Practice. Repetition and practice are the keys to mastery. When you're practicing, you're expanding your comfort zone. Practice AACV at least twice per day. Practice affirmations once per day. Institute scenario practice regularly, according to the schedule. Be engaged in the conversation and in the community on a regular basis.

Step 15: Share. Find a way to be the teacher or lead someone to the teachings. The teacher always learns more than the student. Helping another helps you practice and stay engaged.

Appendix A: Online POP Resources
In Order of Appearance

Share your Story. Readers share their stories of viewing and doing addiction and recovery, www.poweroverpornography.com/shareyour-story

Commitment letter, poweroverpornography.com/commitment

Calendar (personalized course schedule), poweroverpornography.com/calendar

Consequences research, poweroverpornography.com/consequences

Vision development and sharing, poweroverpornography.com/vision

Preformatted AACV card, poweroverpornography.com/AACVcard

Rationalizations used by viewers, poweroverpornography.com/rationalizations

Help with affirmations, poweroverpornography.com/affirmations

Help with relationships, poweroverpornography.com/relationships

Help with scenarios for scenario practice, poweroverpornography.com/scenarios

Practice program and schedule, poweroverpornography.com/practice

Forums: what's working for other POP clients, answers to your questions, getting help if you need it, poweroverpornography.com/forums

Spiritual principles, poweroverpornography.com/spiritualprinciples

Online course, poweroverpornography.com/course

Other Resources (not included in text of book):

Current Articles, including videos, poweroverpornography.com/articles

Free CD of a Brian Brandenburg interview discussing the keys to success using the Power over Pornography program, poweroverpornography.com/freecd

Newsletter list: a monthly e-mail newsletter to keep you in the discussion of Power over Pornography and living the life of love. Keeps you updated on the latest research and findings, poweroverpornography.com/newsletter

Links to valuable resources outside of the POP family: poweroverpornography.com/links

In Order of Appearance

POP: Power over Pornography. The name of this program to help you overcome your addiction to pornography and/or masturbation.

Viewing (V): The act of viewing pornography in any of its forms.

Viewer: Pornography addict, viewer of pornography.

Doing (D): The act of masturbating.

Doer: A person who masturbates.

Living a Loving Life or **Living a Life of Love:** Living a life free of pornography viewing and free of masturbation. Overcoming pornography and masturbation addictions or habits results in an increased capacity to love and increased happiness derived from close relationships.

Cloudy or **Cloudiness:** This refers to long-term consequences being less clear than short-term consequences and how they will become less clear with time unless we deliberately bring them to the front of our minds or, in other words, erase their cloudiness.

Rule of Five: When you select more than five goals, your focus becomes too diffuse to accomplish them. By limiting your goals, lists, or focus to five or fewer items, you increase your chances of success.

MuHa: Must or have to. The use of this or other compulsory language takes away your freedom to choose. When you hear yourself say it, correct it by letting out a "Muhaha" laugh.

BOSS: Better, ought to, should, and supposed to. This is more compulsory language. When you use any of these words, you empower them to become your boss instead of taking the power back from them.

AACV: Acknowledge and accept the temptation, exercise your freedom to choose, and choose your vision. This is the essence of POP.

SAD: Stress, anxiety and discomfort. When you view and do to escape SAD, SAD becomes stronger and larger. Embrace the SAD you may feel when you start the program and realize that you are changing for the better and enlarging your comfort zone.

SAPS: Suppress, avoid, protect, and substitute. These are the common paths to overcoming pornography that typically fail. Whenever you find yourself doing any of the following, it's time to get back on the AACV program: Suppress the temptation, avoid triggers and temptations, rely upon external protection, and substitute another thought or action. Otherwise, you are headed for relapse.

RAACV: Recognize the temptation, acknowledge it, accept it, and choose your vision. "Recognize" is added to the AACV process when traveling and in circumstances when new or unexpected temptations arise.

Thank you for reading!

Dear Reader,

I hope you enjoyed Power Over Pornography and that it is having a positive impact on your life. I've received many letters from fellow readers like you thanking me for the book. Some described the steps that helped them the most while others offered some suggestions.

As an author, I love feedback. I incorporated some of it in the latest edition and would love to hear from you. Tell me what you liked, what helped you the most, even what was least helpful. You can write me at my personal email address, bkbranden@gmail.com and visit me on the web at poweroverpornography.com.

Finally, I need to ask a favor. If you're so inclined, I'd love a review of Power Over Pornography. Reviews can be tough to come by these days. You, the reader, have the power to make or break a book. By providing a review, you help the book get discovered by others who can begin living a loving life. If you have the time, here is a link to my author page on Amazon: http://www.amazon.com/Brian-Brandenburg/e/B008SZ44R4.

Thank you for reading Power Over Pornography and for spending time with me.

In gratitude,

Brian Brandenburg

[i.] This quote is most often loosely attributed to Carl Jung but other sources list L. Ron Hubbard as the originator.

[ii.] David O. McKay, Conference Report, Apr. 1950, p. 32.

[iii.] Patrick Carnes, *Don't Call It Love*.

[iv.] Mark H. Butler, "Is There Hope for a Pornography Addiction?" The Digital Universe, February 7, 2013.

[v.] Patrick Carnes, *Don't Call It Love*.

Made in United States
North Haven, CT
04 June 2023

37340735R00111